A Double-Edged Life

*A memoir of a young woman's journey
with bipolar*

JILL GEBHART CAMPBELL

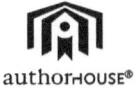

authorHOUSE®

AuthorHouse™
1663 Liberty Drive
Bloomington, IN 47403
www.authorhouse.com
Phone: 1-800-839-8640

First published by AuthorHouse 8/11/2009

ISBN: 978-1-4389-8089-8 (e)
ISBN: 978-1-4389-8087-4 (sc)
ISBN: 978-1-4389-8088-1 (hc)

Printed in the United States of America
Bloomington, Indiana

This book is printed on acid-free paper.

The collage on the front cover was created during a manic episode: a witch's brew of feelings, fears, and a combination of manic thoughts—thoughts that rise above normalcy and plunge to the depths of human despair.

Table of Contents

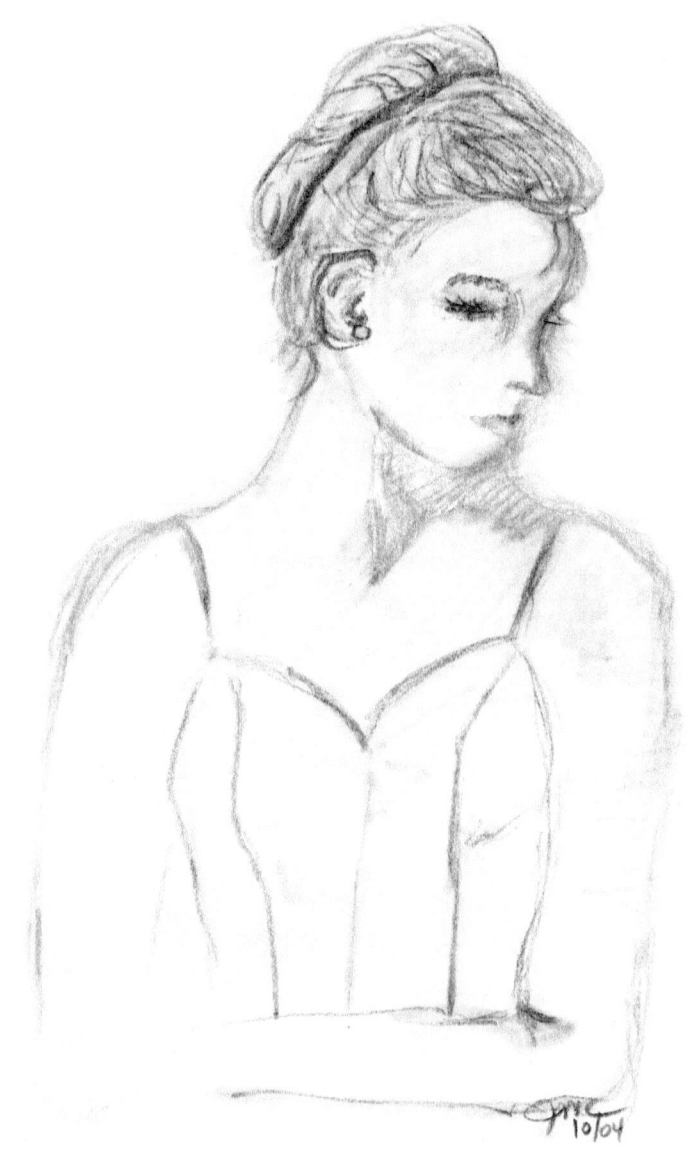

Jill Campbell (Ebony Pencil)

Gazing through the window my soul
Escapes the confines of reality
Refracting images of me
Perceptions stand still

I dedicate this book to my mother, my father, and my best friend and twin sister, Kristin, who helped see me through this. My children, Brandon and Kayla, who have brought such joy to our lives. Gloria, who spent endless amounts of time editing this book. Dr. Clark, who saved me from myself. But especially to my husband, who lived it.

To Dan~
You bring calmness upon the waves
Peace you sing to me amidst the billows
I breathe easier with you by my side

Introduction

This book is a reflection of how the devastating effects of bipolar disorder have shaped my life. It is also reflective of loved ones who have endured the pain of this illness with me. Friends and family have had extraordinary compassion and healing in their wings. My husband has exercised tolerance far beyond the seemingly possible. My dad believed I could be anything I wanted to be, and my mother showed unconditional love and unfailing compassion. I have suffered seventeen years of depression and mania, which distorted my vision of the world in which I live and robbed me at times of a sense of reality and sanity. However, I've come to a realization that God still lives, despite our suffering, and He has been present yesterday and is present today.

My passion for poetry, writing, and art prompted me to write a book including these creative genres in order to portray my bipolar illness in a more personal way. Written expression has been an outlet to purge myself from bitterness and from this enemy that seems to be so relentless and so unconquerable. Keeping a journal has enabled me to recollect memories from both before and after the diagnosis, events and feelings I would never have been able to recall. My twin sister, Kristin, has also contributed material, as have doctors. My attempt to tell the whole story will be with honesty and integrity in order to help and encourage others who contend with this shattering disease and have faced its demons in their own lives. My failures and successes have helped me to better understand humanity as I reflect on this journey and on those who have walked with me. I hope and pray that in some way my journey will help carry you through yours.

Foreword:

The Nature of Bipolar

"...the swallowing gulf of dark forgetfulness and deep oblivion."

~William Shakespeare, *Richard III*

Bipolar disorder almost succeeded in pushing me over the edge. It seeped into every facet of my life, every part of my being, requiring a life-changing perspective on how I thought I would live my life.

Although bipolar disorder is a physical condition, I am always acutely aware of the mental illness stigma. When people find out I'm bipolar, I get this sense of myself as smeared on the slide of a microscope. The accompanying paranoia is equally damaging to my soul. It is perhaps the most embarrassing and degrading aspect of my disorder.

I never knew whom I could trust. After baring the most private parts of my life, I would end up feeling extremely paranoid and worthless. It was debilitating. And frightening. I lost confidence in myself as well as my trust in others—even close family members and friends. I've suffered seventeen years from this cruel illness and have finally found relief after taking myself off of Lithium, the drug commonly used to treat bipolar. My replacement medication has been stabilized for almost a year, and I've found my exuberance for life returning.

Bipolar, also known as manic depressive illness, is a physical disease that afflicts 5.7 million people in the United States, approximately 2.6 percent of adults. It affects both men and women equally. People between the ages of 15 and 25 have the greatest risk of developing this disorder. It is estimated that some form of mental illness affects one in five families in America.[1]

"Bipolar disorder is…defined by the presence of one or more episodes of abnormally elevated mood clinically referred to as mania or, if milder, hypomania. Individuals who experience manic episodes also commonly experience depressive episodes or symptoms, or mixed episodes in which features of both mania and depression are present at the same time."[2] These episodes are triggered by stress—such as overwork, loss of job, family problems, difficult relationships, illness, or negative life events.

Some of the major symptoms of mania include elevated levels of energy, grandiose ideas, racing and confused thoughts, increased irritability, and impulsive activities. Most often, those who experience mania are not able to see their behavior as abnormal. They believe they have more energy and may feel on the "high" side of life—highly efficient, successful, energetic, and creative. Mania may lead to other, unwanted, behaviors: hallucinations, both auditory and visual; anxiety; hostility; obsessive/compulsive behavior; as well as dangerous and erratic behavior. Conversely, depression results in excessive or diminished sleep patterns, suicidal thinking, pessimism, poor concentration, and/or loss of memory.

"The exact causes of mental disorders are still widely unknown; however, most specialists believe they are likely caused by multiple factors interacting together to create a chemical imbalance in certain areas of the brain."[1] Neurotransmitters (chemicals released in the brain) are essential to proper brain functioning; if these chemicals are too high or too low, they may cause bipolar symptoms—either elevated or depressed states. Genetics is also a factor.

One of the difficulties in diagnosing bipolar illness is the need to distinguish it from other conditions that frequently overlap mood disorders. Having bipolar seems to make one more vulnerable to other anxiety ailments such as alcoholism and substance abuse, panic disorder, bulimia, attention deficit disorder, and migraine headaches. These are almost always improved by the successful treatment of bipolar.

Instead of viewing mental illness as a physical disease—such as diabetes, arthritis, or high blood pressure—many people see it as a personal weakness due to poor intellect, lack of character, or socioeconomic factors. "Just as diabetes is a disorder of the pancreas, mental illnesses are medical conditions that often result in a diminished capacity for coping with the ordinary demands of life."[1] This mental illness stigma not only impacts the way a bipolar person views himself, but it also makes many people uncomfortable.

The greatest risk in bipolar disorder is failure to receive treatment. Many individuals may refuse treatment because of denial, lack of information, the stigma associated with mental illness, or an inability to pay for medication. Without treatment the episodes escalate, often resulting in the compromise of careers, relationships, finances, and overall health. Untreated people suffer higher death rates from suicide, heart disease, or strokes. It is imperative that a person with bipolar accept that he has a mental illness and monitor shifts in mood and behavior.

Another difficulty in maintaining proper treatment is that people with bipolar disorder often have natural periods of remission, but without treatment they will relapse. Perhaps they think they are cured; bipolar, however, does not go away.

Although living with any type of mental illness is difficult, those who suffer from bipolar experience shame, hopelessness, and worthlessness. These feelings can generally be improved with psychotherapy and medication, as well as a healthy lifestyle—exercise, regular sleep, and proper eating habits—which leads to a more stable life. In addition, an enjoyable career, sport, or hobby can contribute to feelings of self-worth. Positive thinking and healthy relationships can be highly beneficial in the recovery process. It is important to hold onto the affirmation that life can return to normality, particularly if one is vigilant in observing stressors that contribute to manic and depressive states.

Fortunately, this mystifying disorder is both treatable and manageable with the proper dosage of medication, counseling, and the strategies and skills to deal with traumatic episodes. "The best treatments for serious mental illness are highly successful; between 70 and 90 percent of individuals have significant reduction of symptoms and improved quality of life with a combination of pharmacological and psychosocial treatments and support."[1] Strategies that have helped me include creative expression in artwork, poetry, or writing; keeping a journal; and seeking spiritual guidance. My journal-keeping has enabled me to chart my changes in mood, energy, and behavior. Tracking these changes enables me to see the patterns in my behavior and has served as an indicating factor that my medication regimen is working effectively. These indicators have helped me and my doctor develop a long-term plan for maintaining and improving my mental health.

Without support, solving problems and dealing with the challenges that accompany any mental illness can seem utterly overwhelming. Several bipolar support groups are available, as well as websites that provide information and insight into bipolar illness. Associations such as the National Alliance for Mental Illnesses (NAMI), World Health Organization (WHO), and the Depression Bipolar Support

Alliance (DBSA) offer support to those affected by this disorder, as well as support to their loved ones.

It is imperative that people are informed correctly about the devastating effects of bipolar illness. Not enough is being done to educate society that bipolar is a physical disease that is highly treatable with the correct dosage of medication. "Simply put, treatment works, if you can get it. But in America today, it is clear that many people living with the most serious and persistent mental illnesses are not provided with the essential treatment they need."[3] As a result, society bears the overwhelming burden of paying for hospitalizations, disability, unemployment, suicide, and incarceration that stem from this illness.

It is my hope that understanding this illness will not only help the person who has bipolar, but educate society and loved ones who are affected by it.

1. National Alliance on Mental Illness. Accessed May 26, 2009, http://www. nami.org/Content/NavigationMenu/Inform_Yourself/About_Mental_ Illness/About_Mental_Illness.htm and http://www.nami.org/Template. cfm?Section=About_Mental_Illness&Template=/ContentManagement/ ContentDisplay.cfm&ContentID=53155.

2. http://Wikipedia.org/wiki/Bipolar-disorder. Accessed May 26, 2009.

3. National Alliance on Mental Illness. (2006). Grading the states: A report on America's health care system for serious mental illness: Arlington, VA.

CHAPTER ONE

A Promising Beginning

"There is nothing more helpful in life than a good remembrance,
particularly a remembrance from our childhood, when we still
lived in our parents' home."

~Fyodor Dostoyevsky, *The Brothers Karamazov*

The following memories are significant in trying to reconstruct my life before the onset of the illness at age twenty-one. I had the benefit of an exceptionally wonderful childhood. My mom and dad were greatly supportive and instrumental in helping Kristin and me build confidence in ourselves and in our athletic and academic abilities.

In 1976, when Kristin and I were six, my dad stood outside all night long pumping water into our sandbox, half the size of a basketball court. He stayed out there in sub zero degree weather while the water turned into ice to make a hockey rink. It took him an entire week to completely freeze the sand box. Every morning when the snow settled on the rink he would go outside and shovel it so we could skate and play hockey. We started skating on double runner skates. When my dad saw that we were falling all the time, he decided we needed helmets. He also bought knee and elbow pads, hockey sticks, and a puck. Thus began our love for and proficiency in sports.

About the same time that we learned hockey, we also began to enjoy another sport, football. We watched Denver's football team on Sundays and on the occasional Monday night, cheering as John Elway led the Broncos to the Super Bowl. During football games, my dad, my sister, and I invented a tickle game. We ran around our dad, while he laid on the floor and tried to catch us by our legs. If he caught us, we'd get tickled.

Several years later, in 1981, we traveled regularly from Denver to other cities, including Colorado Springs—over an hour and a half drive—to play competitive soccer. Our parents were, of course, our biggest fans. We spent many weekends playing in tournaments, both instate and out of state.

In 1984, Kristin and I made the high-school varsity soccer team as freshmen. We played on varsity for the remainder of our high-school careers. During this time, after passing the rigorous all-day tryouts at the Air Force Academy in Colorado Springs, we played on a state select team and traveled with the team to various states.

In July 1987, Kristin was selected to go to China with the Colorado National Women's Soccer Team. I was asked to join the team when the coach's daughter cancelled. We left Denver for a twenty-one-hour plane ride to China. During our flight we had a difficult time conversing with the stewardess, although she was most helpful in assisting us with our paperwork. After we arrived at customs, we had another flight for two more hours.

We played in front of crowds of 30,000 or more. It was thrilling, even though I hardly played. Kristin was instrumental on the team. Our first game we won 4–0. Although I only played the last fifteen minutes of the game, I didn't mind; I was fascinated with Chinese culture and the people. The coaches kept getting us confused. At the end of the game, one of the coaches came up to me and said, "Outstanding game, Kristin," and I smilingly replied, "Thanks, but I'm not Kristin!"

We had memorable scenic tours. On our first tour we went to the Summer Palace, where intricate ceiling paintings spanned miles of walkway. I became caught up in the different culture and lifestyle. The people had a lower standard of living, but they seemed enviably happy and very hospitable. They prepared banquets in every city we toured. On one occasion, they organized a dance, lining up chairs all around the dance floor with Christmas lights strung across the ceiling. The girls danced with each other during the slow dances. I loved the people in this country; they were very family-oriented and kind. They had what are now considered "old-fashioned" values.

The behavior of one group of American girls was very embarrassing. They became drunk and were rude, obnoxious, and disrespectful. These girls portrayed the United States poorly. It was distressing to me because many of the Chinese think all Americans are lacking in courtesy and spoiled. In addition to the previous rude behavior, two girls set off the fire extinguisher while staying at the hotel. They said that they wanted to have a water fight. The Chinese people were yelling and running all over the place; they got out their vacuums at two in the morning to clean it up. They did not think it was funny. I didn't either; I was so ashamed for my country. During the final game, three of our girls got into a fist fight with three of the Chinese players. Some of the girls on our team were using vulgar signs and language. I was never so embarrassed as I was then.

One night after ten o'clock in the evening, several of us sat outside the hotel talking and reading scriptures in the median that divided the road. Two boys came up and started speaking Chinese to us. We wanted to tell them about Christ but we were unable to have a conversation. It was then that I realized how important it was to communicate, and I desperately wanted to understand them. How I wished that I could speak a little Chinese! We couldn't converse

3

so they left. We sat up until 11:30 that night, watching the people. Many families slept on the sidewalks with nowhere else to lay their heads, and other people wandered the streets at night without shelter and with little food. I thought a lot about the people and their feelings; I wondered if the people hated communism and blamed their poverty on the government. From my perspective they were poor in body but rich in spirit. Art, architecture, poetry, religion, and history were embedded with high morals in these people. This trip would inspire me to study Chinese in college, with the hope that someday I would return and serve as a missionary in China.

On the third night in Beijing, I knelt down and prayed on the dirty floor in our hotel. I felt close to God in this beautiful land, where the people seemed so pure and undefiled.

I learned on bended knee
He was a reality
His blood He freely spilt
Erasing my everlasting guilt
Tears I shed yesterday
Prayers I prayed today
Christ heard my gentle plea
I learned on bended knee

We also visited several tourist sites from Diamond Lake, including the Yangtze River (formerly the Yellow River—the beautiful sand and silt make the river look yellow) and, most impressive, The Great Wall. The wall took centuries to build and creates a barrier over 6,000 miles long, snaking over hills, mountains, and plains to keep the Mongolians from invading China. The towers on the wall served as vantage points to view an impending invasion. Reflecting on this today, I realize that the view from the tower of my life would be obscured as I fought my own personal enemy.

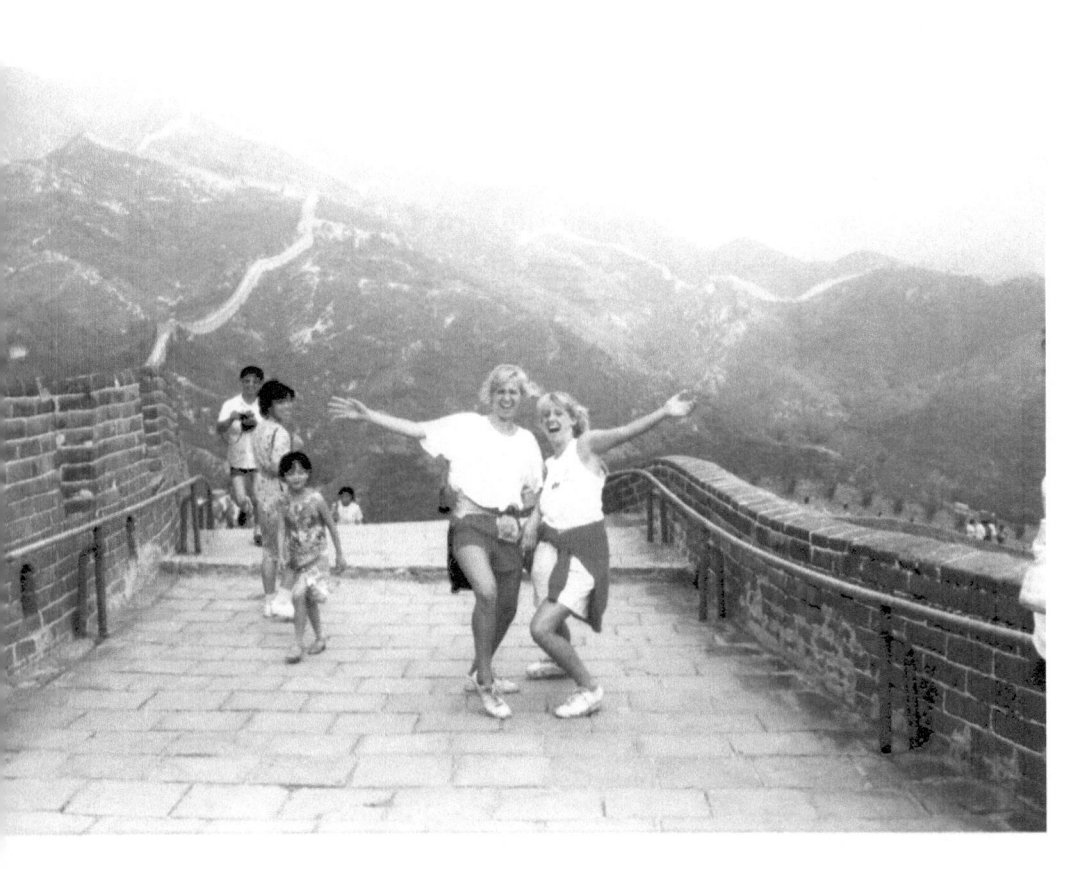

Twins on Great Wall
July 1987

Upon my return to America three weeks later, I had never felt so alone. Forests of buildings, concrete walls, empty streets, and flashing lights replaced simplicity and the natural beauty of dirt streets and fire pits to light up the night life. I found myself missing the serenity and sincerity of the Chinese people, for whom I have never lost the love that was fostered on that visit. China was the highlight of my life, and I was never the same.

~~~~~~~~~~~~~~~~~~~~~

During my senior year, as a way to find comfort during an episode of depression, I spent a lot of time reading scriptures, writing poetry, seeking strength through spiritual enlightenment, and listening to worship music. I also discovered a new passion in art that allowed me to express myself in another way. I drew the following self-portrait that year.

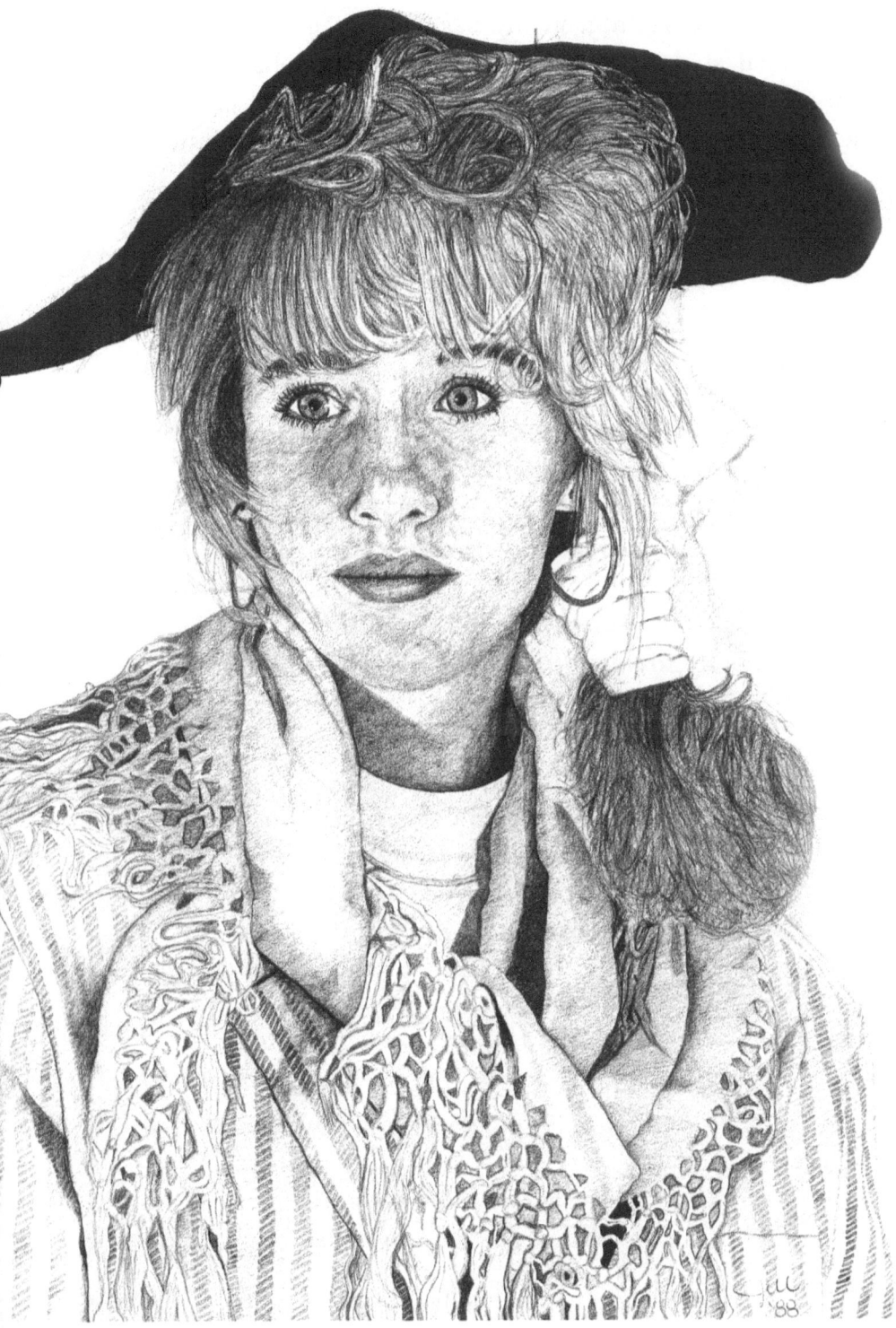

I hoped that these outlets would somehow rescue me from my depression. Reflecting on my past, I realize that I was highly emotional at age fifteen and zealous about religion. Although this poem was written in college before the onset of my illness, it expresses perfectly my profound love and understanding that I feel for my Savior.

Christ the child's birth set us free
His crowning act suffered in Gethsemane
Tears like rain poured freely
As our Savior was crucified on a tree

God and Christ created a plan
To redeem all who would stand
Our hearts groaned within
As His blood poured for man's sin

Skies were rent with black
As sinners thrashed whips into his back
He carried His cross 'til He could no more
Upon Calvary, our cross He bore

He descended below the least of man
Miracles preceding His earthly plan
His life that He freely gave to all
Would ransom man from the fall

Will He ever know of my love?
Following Him to courts above
Do His will, praise His name
Embrace charity, forego fame

To see with the Savior's eyes
To witness His eternal sunrise

Brighter than the eastern star
Make me worthy of it all

The following journal entry was written at age eighteen. I was consumed by religion and world peace. Today I realize that the reality of Jesus Christ and the spirituality I feel today when reading the Bible was not part of the religious fanaticism that I experienced during my diagnosis.

My words found access above
God heard my eager plea
Willing me to hear His love
He sent Christ to me
He must have known
He saved my soul
Until His love was shown
My heart was dark as coal
Although I know you accept me
Sometimes I stumble and fall
I imagine sitting at your knee
Am I worthy of it all?

Journal entry:
In this decade nuclear threat was and is a reality. I remember at the age of fourteen watching a television program, "The Day After." The show was about nuclear reaction and the effects that radiation would have on the globe. I remember the fear I felt watching the show. That night, I fell asleep with tears rolling onto my pillow. I was frightened. At school the next day, that's all we talked about.

The Persian Gulf crisis seems to be escalating. Everything keeps getting worse. The United Nations has passed sanctions for us to go to war. Why can't we live in harmony and peace within our souls—every man, woman, and child?

~~~~~~~~~~~~~~~~~~~~~~~

In 1987 Kristin and I began our senior year of high school. We started cross country and were instrumental in Student Government. Kristin made the honor roll every semester during high school. We had a small business selling lollipops and servicing revolving lollipops stands at local convenience stores. My good friend Heather Gifford and I conducted a seminar for the freshman class called, "The greatest days of our lives." And they were great times; never did I guess at the ominous dark clouds looming large on the horizon for me. Toward the end of September, I worked on the Air Band with the student council. We were also spending our days in the Post Graduate Center. BYU was my number one choice for college. The student council retreat was coming up, and we were preparing the packet for the retreat. It was a hectic time.

Kristin applied to University of Denver and Colorado College with the dream of playing on a division one soccer team; however, because I applied to Brigham Young University, she put in an application as well. After being accepted to BYU, Kristin, with reservations, decided that we would attend BYU together. We had the expectation that we would be roommates because we were each other's greatest support and pushed each other to excel in academics and athletics. At that time, BYU didn't have a division one soccer team with scholarships, so we played on the club team. Today, Kristin says, "I can't look back; it breaks my heart not to have played for a division one soccer team."

Kristin and I packed our bags in August and with our dad headed to Provo, Utah, to attend college at Brigham Young University. We traveled through Glenwood Canyon, where they were building an overpass on Interstate 70. We spent a few hours waiting for our turn to proceed. During the long wait, Kristin and I went for a run along the mountain road; the mountains had a serenity about them, and it was extremely peaceful . We returned and stretched. The trip was long, and I passed much of the time reading. I read a book titled *Life and Death in Shanghai* about the atrocities the Chinese people endured during the Cultural Revolution. Many people were under house arrest due to the corrupt leadership of Mao Zedong. After being in China and witnessing the beauty of that country, I couldn't imagine the immense suffering they had endured.

A few years later, on my way home from classes, I saw a Chinese lady crying in front of the Clyde Engineering Building on the southeast side of the BYU campus. Her distress was so obvious that I stopped to ask her why she was crying. With what little English she knew and the small amount of Chinese I had, HanQi and I seemed to understand one another. She told me that her son DiDi (Andy) was failing the sixth grade because he didn't know any English. That morning Andy was supposed to graduate from the sixth grade, and the principal told HanQi that he would not graduate. They made him sit on the side of the room while the other children participated in singing and graduation ceremonies. This was extremely humiliating and heartbreaking for her because she had a PhD in Mechanical Engineering and was teaching at BYU. As I walked home with her, she told me that Andy had run away. I helped her find him; he was playing on the swings and in the mud. He had mud caked all over his arms, legs, ears, and face. He was a chubby ten-year-old boy with porcelain skin. I said hello to him in Chinese and spoke a few sentences to him.

Afterward, we went inside her modest apartment, where she gave me strawberry ice cream while Andy cleaned up. I took him outside to play soccer and showed him how to play goalie, and he taught me a few words in Chinese. His mother came out and took pictures of us heading the ball back and forth. She noticed that Andy seemed to forget all about the sadness he had felt about not graduating earlier that day.

We went back inside and HanQi prepared Chinese food, which we all ate together. Andy was excited to show me pinyin (Chinese words in English). I told him that I would come play with him and we could teach each other Chinese and English. Andy's mother came over and hugged me with tears in her eyes and told me that "the gods had arranged our meeting." I agreed. I told her that we would be good friends and that I would teach Andy English. For an hour every day, for over a year, I taught him how to speak and read English. They are beautiful people. When I left for Ontario, California, for the summer, I gave him a notebook that I made with writing activities, and we corresponded via mail. He would enter the seventh grade more proficient in English.

I maintained contact with Andy and his mother. Years later, he would apply to several universities. He wrote his college entrance paper, "Who was the most influential person in your life?" about me. He was accepted to the University of Buffalo in Buffalo, New York, where he finished his undergraduate degree in engineering and then earned a master's degree at GeorgiaTech in Atlanta in design engineering. It was a pleasure for me to watch his progress and success and to be involved with this Chinese family. I love them dearly.

~~~~~~~~~~~~~~~~~~~~~

Just as in high school, I played goalkeeper at BYU and led the team to many scoreless games. Kristin played center halfback and was consistently a top scorer. Our team traveled in two twelve-passenger vans both to California and Colorado every fall to compete against other teams. When our team was in Denver, we played the University of Denver, Colorado State University, and the University of Colorado at Boulder. Our parents hosted the Brigham Young soccer team whenever we were in town. Dad would cook three pounds of spaghetti and bake five loaves of garlic bread for these parties. In the morning, he made eggs, bacon, and toast. The team stayed overnight several nights and slept wall to wall in our house.

Road trips were especially enlivening. Not only did we develop close relationships, we had lots of laughs and made lasting memories. On Fisherman's Wharf in San Francisco, we walked along the wharf, ate clam chowder, shopped, and listened to a blues singer who had his guitar case open to put money in for the entertainment.

We also ran. Kristin ran the New York Marathon in 1990 and placed second in her age group. I ran the St. George Marathon with Julie Anderson, one of my best friends and a college roommate, and placed second in my weight category. Two years later, Kristin would walk onto BYU's division one cross-country team, where she ran consistently in the top seven runners. The integral part sports played in my life probably kept me in the physical shape I needed to endure the destructive upheavals that were to come my way.

On one occasion in December of 1988, during our freshman year in college, Kristin and I went running at two o'clock in the morning. Snow fell gently, snowflakes resting on our heads. The moonlight made the snow glisten. The trail was uncharted and pristine until we left our footprints on the virgin snow. It was wonderfully peaceful—our feet rhythmically pounding on the powdered snow, our shoulders touching ever so slightly with each step. The silence of the night permeated our senses with every breath, words not spoken in the isolation of the night.

Unknown to me, that would be my most peaceful memory for a long time.

An Accumulation of Stress

"For weeks the truth had hung on the edge of consciousness, but she had turned from it with the heart's instinctive clinging to the unrealities by which it lives."

~Edith Wharton, *The Custom of the Country*

During my off-season from soccer in 1990, I coached a soccer team and taught physical education at Meridian Middle School. It was there that I experienced a significant physical injury. A poorly designed, handcrafted soccer goalpost weighing over 200 pounds was not well-secured to the ground, and it fell over on my legs during a wind storm. As the wind blew the post over, the girls on the field were yelling at me to run forward but it was too late, the goalpost clipped my legs. I was lucky that it did not fall in a more vital place.

I was lying in the emergency room for quite some time. The nurses were unable to give me pain killers without a doctor's permission, and the pain was intense. Kristin was crying and told me to "look over to my side so I know you're all right." She saw how deformed my legs were and was terribly frightened. I had to make a private joke so she would laugh through her tears, but I knew when she looked at my legs she was scared. My bones weren't broken but the pole had damaged the muscles in my legs and compressed the skin to the bone making my legs look abnormally thin. It was truly frightening not to have any feeling in my legs for more than three days; I dreaded the thought that I might be paralyzed. When feeling returned to my legs I woke up almost every hour in severe pain and prayed that I would be able to walk again. Kristin and my roommate Jennifer stayed up all night with me for nights on end.

The second day of therapy, Gary, the physical therapist, rubbed my legs in an attempt to push the blood to my upper body. It was extremely painful. After three weeks, I still had hemorrhaging in my lower legs where my calf muscle had been flattened. The bar made an impression on my right calf where it had impacted my leg. Shane, another therapist, was afraid I had damaged the muscles in my lower legs; however, the MRI found nothing wrong with the muscles. Walking was an impossibility, and I lived on the third floor. A man who lived in the same apartment building carried me upstairs. After several weeks, I could walk with crutches. I couldn't walk without them for what seemed like an endless time. Shane and I spent many days on the hospital lawn where I did forward and backward sprints in order to rehabilitate my legs. Although I continued coaching the girl's team I couldn't stand for more than five minutes at a time.

Because I kept falling I was afraid that I wouldn't be able to play soccer that fall. I had the entire summer to strengthen my legs, and in my determination to heal I started walking up the side of "Y" mountain, a switchback hill above my apartment building. Eventually strength returned to my legs, and I was able to play soccer in the fall. However, the results of the injury are still present and my legs go numb every day. To this day I have an impression on my leg the width of the bar. I thank God that I can walk.

When I returned home for fall break of 1990, my mom rubbed the blood in my legs to my upper body and stroked my hair. Her reassurance gave me comfort beyond the imaginable. I spent many days with my head in her lap. My mother is a saint, and I love her dearly. Her compassion toward me is indicative of the way she has lived her life. She is an avid reader, enjoys gardening, and makes beautiful clothing and quilts. Her involvement in book clubs, Bunko, and outings with friends keep her engaged with the lives of others. While I was suffering from my manic and depressive episodes she was instrumental in keeping a stable environment for our children while Dan worked. Much of her time with our children was spent playing games, working puzzles and reading. She is a strong advocate for education and has influenced our children to excel in academics. She has been a blessing in the lives of so many people!

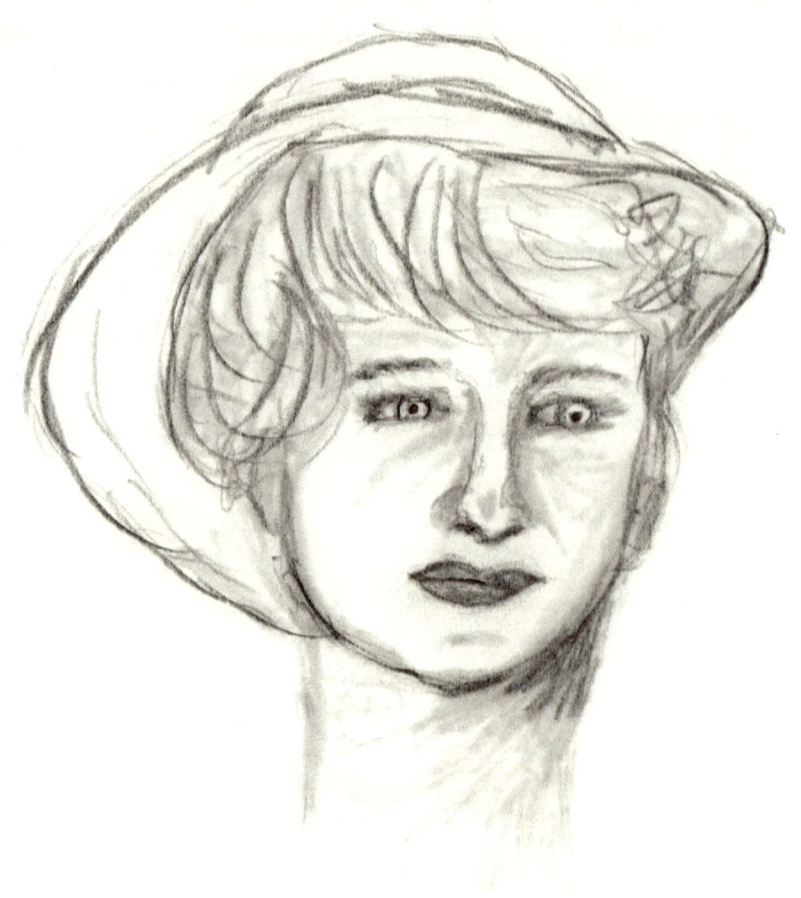

Ame
11/04

Like a tapestry created by God's hand
The threads of your character
Weave colors into my life

My life before the onset of bipolar illness was exciting and adventuresome. During the summer of 1990, my best friend Jennifer, her brother Jason, and I traveled by car to the East Coast. Kristin went to Camp Echo Lake, a Jewish camp in upstate New York, to work as a camp counselor. We traveled hours out of our way to visit her. I missed her terribly. This was the longest time we had ever been apart. On our way we slept at rest stops, sleeping both in and out of our car, sometimes waking up with dew on the grass. We visited several Universities, including Columbia, Dartmouth, Boston University, and my favorite, Harvard. In Washington D.C. we walked along the Mall, watched People to People (a dance and singing group), and spent the Fourth of July on the lawn outside the Washington D.C. monument with thousands of other people. In Boston, we rode our mountain bikes along the Charles River and ate at hole-in-the-wall restaurants. We had a memorable summer!

The summer of 1991 brought many stresses, as well as some high points. I traveled to Ontario, California, with my best friend Julie to teach English to exchange students from Japan and Spain. The man we were working for required us to find homes where these students could stay at no cost. We knocked on doors for days without any success. When the students arrived, we had no curriculum, and each day we made up different worksheets and taught from various workbooks. We didn't have any formal training for teaching English as a second language. We were required to take the students on outings to Disneyland and other tourist sites.

On one of these, in Los Angeles, Julie and I met a beautiful homeless woman named Elizabeth. She had been living on the streets for some time and had been struck by a bus three weeks earlier. I had just purchased a new pair of tennis shoes, which I promptly returned so I could give Elizabeth the money. Julie and I told her how much we loved her. Her black coal-colored eyes collected pools of tears as they fell from her lovely face and she told us, "Do you know how long it's been since someone told me that they loved me?"

We hugged her again and held her in our arms for what seemed like several minutes. She said the only way she made it on the streets is that she knew Jesus Christ loved her. We hugged her again and tears rolled down my cheeks as I watched Elizabeth hobble down the street with forty dollars in her pocket and her faith in the Savior.

As we were teaching the Japanese students English, Bruce Douglas walked into the church. He was dressed in a gas-attendant uniform; his skin was jet black, and his hair was greased back in a disorderly fashion. His face was dim, his mouth stretched downward by discouragement—but his eyes shone brightly. He motioned his hand with his palm facing upward, encouraging me to approach him. I couldn't ignore the eager look on this gentleman's face, so I left the students and introduced myself to him. He stammered, telling me that, "Since this is a church and all, maybe someone could help me out?" He hadn't been able to find a job for months and needed only ten dollars to get on a bus to San Francisco.

I told Bruce that if he would help me teach English for a few hours I would give him the money he needed to pay for the bus fare. He agreed, and I had him stand in front of the class as each student looked directly at Bruce and told him his name. I don't think Bruce had ever had so much attention in his life. He hadn't received a very good education and had trouble reading in the class, but with some encouragement he went around to the students pointing out different words in English. His eyes became even brighter, and he began to smile. Julie gave him some money to get something to eat.

He came back fifteen minutes later, and we continued class. We went outside on the lawn. Bruce passed out the music, and we sang "I Am a Child of God" while Julie played the guitar. After we finished singing, we gave Bruce twenty dollars and bid him good-bye. Through his teary eyes, he said, "I'm going to be a teacher, I'm going to school." I told him that Christ loves him and that he could be anything he wanted. His eyes flashed with determination at me as he said, "I will make a difference." Little did he know that he already had made a difference in our lives. A week later, we received a phone call from Bruce. He said he was entering school and needed money for tuition. Julie and I sent him 100 dollars to get on his feet.

After several weeks of not getting paid from the man who ran the ESL program, we decided it was time to hunt him down. We scouted him out at a nearby hotel where we confronted him. He assured us that we would get our money. However, it would be several more weeks before we did, and it was much less than the amount we had negotiated. The fee for the program was exorbitant, and he had squandered most of the money.

We weren't getting enough sleep, and I became ill with a fever of 102 degrees. We had no backups, and it required two of us to handle the students. The three stressful months we spent teaching and taking students on tours weakened the links that held the chain of my mental health.

I tell these stories for a specific reason, to remember that before the onset of my illness I was a kind, loving, and compassionate young woman. After my diagnosis and eventual weight gain I became self-consumed with little confidence, low self-esteem, and scant capacity to empathize with others.

Julie and I returned to BYU that fall and we began playing soccer in August. My sister and I kept up the grueling schedule that we had begun in high school and added to in college. In the midst of soccer, running, holding a part-time job, coaching, and trips, we did not neglect our studies. Kristin maintained a 3.6 GPA during college, while I held a 3.2. We both majored in humanities with a minor in English and supporting coursework in Chinese and business. Our class loads were heavy.

After soccer practice, we spent almost every night in the library until it closed at midnight. I began feeling depressed and sought counseling from an on-campus professor of psychology, Dr. Gibbons. I would regularly collapse on a couch in his office, exhausted. Among the streams of thoughts I had was a fear that I had different personalities—little girl, bigger girl. He believed me to be schizophrenic and bipolar, but this was an informal diagnosis.

This constant activity and stress had no alternative but to build up to an eruption. Overwhelmed by my class load, studying for hours on end, and holding a part time job, I rarely did anything recreational except for playing soccer and going on the road trips. These trips involved their own kind of stresses, since we missed two days of school, usually Thursday and Friday. That left us with the feeling that we were always needing to "catch up." It was difficult to complete homework while riding in a van with so many distractions. Finally, I began to miss classes and I had a hazy feeling that my thinking wasn't quite right. Stress warnings and red flags seemed to vaguely flicker on the edge of consciousness, but I ignored them. Then my tired body and my stressed and overloaded mind fused into one another and exploded into my illness.

Descent into Darkness

"In a swirling sea, I reach for something solid—but there is only darkness, confusion, and chaos."

~Gloria Reed

The dam finally burst in March 1992. For three weeks, I'd been experiencing psychotic thinking and sleep deprivation. During my continuous waking hours, I spent days and nights mulling over my exam paper in philosophy on Socrates and the Socratic method. Kristin, Julie, Jennifer, and I had just moved from a downstairs apartment to an upstairs apartment in the same building. The original place was still unoccupied so I brought the key, a blanket, pillow, and my book—*The Life and Death of Socrates,* by Plato—so I could be alone.

Socrates said, "Although the unexamined life may not be worth living, the fully examined life cannot be lived." I decided my life was worth examining and I began to feel close to reality itself—although I was completely delusional. In my hallucinations Socrates and I were talking to one another. We stayed up all night, several nights conversing. Socrates had his "head in the clouds" (his expression), and I did too.

Eating became a chore and I rarely showered during this time. I blocked out all distractions and spent several nights isolating myself from Kristin and my roommates. After I turned in my paper about the Sophists, I moved back into my new apartment.

The following day, my roommates left for another day of classes and I was alone with my delusions and inner demons. Unknowingly, I locked myself in my apartment and was convinced that someone else had locked me in. I ran from door to door, window to window in the three-bedroom apartment. I was furiously afraid of the noises I heard and the sights I was seeing—a man with a chainsaw working outside and, simultaneously, a child screaming. I associated these two sounds with each other and felt helpless to save this child from a horrible death. My terror turned to sheer grief as I ran from room to room trying to find a way to rescue the child. Again I ran to the front window, but this time my mind began associating different colors of cars into a pattern. The pattern led me to other windows seeking the next color in the pattern. This hallucination lasted hour after hour, an eternity of endless fright as I waited for my sister to come home.

I called Jennifer at work and urgently warned her not to get into any white vans. Alarmed at my words and the way my voice sounded, she immediately came home. When Julie and my sister arrived, Jennifer insisted that I needed to be hospitalized. Julie and Kristin couldn't accept this. As they debated, I wandered down the stairs. The colors of the cars continued leading me in a whirl of patterns of red, white, and blue. Each color of car told me to follow the next color-coded car. The code color was now blue and it propelled me on my walk. I stopped at a friend's house; she was ironing and the color of water in her spray bottle was blue, so I drank the water. As my journey around the block continued I saw two elderly people, a man and a wife dressed in normal clothes. My visual hallucination made them out to be clownlike. He had blue hair, and she had orange. I was afraid and I started crying.

This would be the beginning of a long descent into darkness and an even longer climb out again.

That evening, Julie and Kristin made a spaghetti dinner for me. It tasted and looked like worms.

> *Lord of Lords*
> *Have you abandoned me?*
> *My eyes don't see clearly*
> *And my heart beats uneasily*
> *If the promise you made me*
> *Years ago, is true*
> *Then why aren't I free*
> *Or am I in bondage to you?*
> *My daily prayers reach upward*
> *But exhausted I can't hear*
> *Though you scream to me*
> *I don't feel you near*

In my next delusion, as is quite common with this illness, I was a hero. If any of the neighbors across from us had their curtains closed, I believed they were "spies" waiting to kill us. I watched for any curtains to close, then went into a frenzy to control the evacuation from the building, warning people about the German tanks that were about to invade us. As I moved from the kitchen window to the front window I stood up on the couch and heard gunshots. I thought that a bullet hit me and I fell to the ground, thinking that my death would save the people from the invasion.

A couple of nights passed; my mania worsened. My sister and Julie were frightened and took me to the emergency room of Utah Valley Community Hospital, where I was eventually admitted to the adult depression unit. Kristin and Julie told them I was acting in an extremely bizarre manner and was difficult to reason with and to manage, that I was crying and then laughing, not sleeping, and making weird and frightening statements about cars and people on the streets. They also said I was afraid I was going to die because of dust in the air and that I didn't want to eat any food because it all had maggots in it.

I was put in a cubicle surrounded by curtains. Julie and Kristin spent the night sleeping next to me in the emergency room on the cold tiled floor, with only a blanket and a pillow. I was hallucinating. I thought the three of us were serving a mission to China and converting the Chinese people to Christianity. I kept passing out and wasn't talking. In the morning, before they transferred me to the psychiatric ward, the lady next to me delivered a baby; I heard a baby cry and in my delusional state I thought I had given birth to the baby and they had taken him away from me. I was devastated and frantic. Ironically, this would prove to be somewhat true with both of my children years later. Both of them were taken immediately to the neonatal intensive care unit as soon as they were born. It would be months before I would be able to hold Kayla and Brandon without tubes.

After admission to the hospital the medical records stated that my chief complaint was, "I don't remember who I am." It further states, "Patient was admitted with rather bizarre symptoms, signing as if deaf and mute, making guttural sounds, not making sense, occasionally breaking into songs." In the morning during transferral to the psychiatric ward on the second floor, I stood on the gurney and belted out John Denver's "Rocky Mountain High" in the elevator. As I was walking down the hall to my room, I went into another patient's room and smashed his guitar. Six staff members tied me down with straps and injected me with medicine to calm me down. Reflecting on my hospitalization, Kristin wrote in her journal: "It was a surreal moment to watch her being admitted. She was a stranger to me both before and during her treatment. My inexperience with bipolar was the greatest blessing of all. Some people say that the unknown is worse than the known. It was best that I didn't know what lay ahead."

Kristin wrote, "I felt locked out from her world as she was locked in it. The door closed on me and I looked only from the outside in. Isolation seemed to be the only way to deal with her major manic episodes. As twins we had always known companionship in having a constant friend in each other; isolation became a dark and lonely memory for both of us."

> *Lonely I sit here thinking thoughts of you*
> *Wondering why our paths seem so divided*
> *Fantasy taking precedence over reality*
> *Why is it I believe in ideas*
> *That become fragmented as time turns*
> *And seasons wear out their welcome*

In order to get an idea of how close our relationship is, one must realize that as identical twins her pain is my pain and my pain is hers. We had our own secret language and enjoyed one another's company above all others. It was difficult to maintain friendships outside of our own. We grew up as "mirrors" of each other. It made this illness even more cruel when Kristin could no longer see her reflection in the "mirror."

> *Reflected in you I see me*
> *Wondering if I see reality*
> *Your godly nature mesmerizes me*
> *Beautiful reflections of me I see*
>
> *Our trails are separate journeys*
> *Surviving on the soul provided me*
> *Memories guide me to eternity*
> *Remembering you, the mirror of me*

Our lives have been parallel in so many ways. It is an intense relationship and one that I greatly cherish. Yet our paths diverged at this point, creating profound loneliness for each of us. Kristin wrote, "They began her treatment, an experimental regimen of drug after drug. All the time, she experienced major effects of the drugs. It continued to separate us further. I felt sick inside."

While I was in the hospital, I had another hallucination that I was in a concentration camp in Germany during the war. I thought I was imprisoned by the Nazis and that there was a secret code among all of the prisoners. This secret code would free us. Doors slamming, lights flickering, and standing inconspicuously by the window were code signals for our escape.

In my room, the windows were barred, the floor and walls were like cement, with the bed in the middle of the floor. The bathrooms were locked and my thirst was unquenchable. The combinations of medicine made me incredibly thirsty and hungry. There was no sink in the locked bathroom and water was given only with meals. The bright overhead light was left on. The following poem expresses perfectly the harsh conditions I existed in and the way it should have been:

The way it should be...
Carpet on the floor
A key for every door
Music to soothe the soul
And a blanket for the cold
Water and food regularly
Release the prisoners
Let their souls free
When you ask me who I am
I might even remember me

During this first hospitalization, Kristin and Julie came often to visit me during my ten-day stay. Julie brought her guitar and we sang songs by John Denver ("Rocky Mountain High") and Dan Fogelberg ("Leader of the Band"). My mom and Kristin brought me blue and white striped shorts and a bright pink top, which I wore every day. My escape was taking frequent showers, where I lathered my body with Neutrogena body oil and my hair with Biolage shampoo. I will never forget the smell of the hospital's coarse towels and washcloths, which smelled like spoiled milk. To this day that odor reminds me of the psychiatric ward. I disliked and distrusted the hospital food but was extremely hungry. We stashed saltine crackers, graham crackers, and juice, so we had something to eat when meals were not served. It was ironic that the food was fattening, and the medicine most of us were on caused us to gain weight.

I felt like I was in "prison" for several years and it turned out I was hospitalized for only twelve days. When I was in a delusional state and my thoughts streamed all around me, time became meaningless. On one occasion I thought I was Amelia Earhart and my plane had crashed and I was imprisoned. I'm not sure how long I was in isolation but it seemed like days before I got water or food. The isolation room smelled like urine and I hated the hospital.

This road I would walk would wind ever uphill. It would be the path I traveled for almost the next two decades of my life. Bipolar illness changed my perspective, and all I could see was the devil beneath the stone and the Son in the skies. So many days I spent crying. My tears flowing freely. Bitterness couldn't get the best of me—I would not let it. When I was able to, I desperately sought a way to escape the pervasive unreality through earnest prayer, good books, artwork, poetry and uplifting music.

> *The Son rises to aid the battered ass*
> *On the blistering path of life*
> *Climbing the terrain of shattered glass*

The Son warms earth dust to suppleness
Nourishing this life of death
Spilling mortality to free bitterness

I spent the nights alone in my room. I felt evil spirits surrounding me, whispering in the silence of the night. I sought refuge in another patient's room after begging the nursing staff for help. I hid underneath the triage center, pleading with them to chase the evil spirits away. They told me to return to my room. I asked them if I could sleep in another room with someone. I felt my way down the dark halls and, overdrugged and without contacts or glasses, the psychiatric unit seemed to have smeared shadows on the walls. I needed to find solace in another room where I might have company against the demons. However, every breath my new roommate took sounded like a gasp for air and once again the evil spirits were tormenting me, and I raced back to my room where my breathing seemed to cut like a knife through the solid air. Nights and days became torturous.

Lonely I am without you
Voices inside talk to me
I stand among
The creatures crazy

Finding your will
To chase away my fear
Evil spirits to kill
Can't anyone hear?

Sleep can't find me
Evading my mind
Inside something's ticking
A bomb with no time.

After a few days, with the help of Haldol (a drug known for calming mania) I swung the other way and became incredibly depressed. Group therapy included confession of your problems to the "group" and sharing stories of obsessive/compulsive and manic/depressive behavior. I walked down the hall to group therapy bumping into walls because I was so drugged. Most of us were so overmedicated by Haldol we couldn't hold our heads up. On many occasions I was so tired and sedated that I'd flop down on my pillow in my room and crawl into bed. I couldn't make it to the group. The staff came to my room, knocked on my door, and demanded that I go to therapy. They wouldn't release me from the hospital until I had "adequate" treatment.

As kindred souls in suffering, we began to develop a camaraderie with one another. The recreational therapy the staff devised for us worked as well as the medicine at times. It consisted of visiting parks to play football and Frisbee and engaging in arts and crafts. The extent of my creativity consisted of pouring different colors of paint in the inside of a coffee mug and swishing it around to coat the inner part of the mug. They thought this was very artistic. Nevertheless it was a nice release from the boredom on the hall; the arts, sports, and music were my only escape from reality.

A friend of mine on the unit recorded a song by Mike and the Mechanics titled, "In the Living Years." The lyrics proved powerful: "It's too late when we die…in the living years." The title is uncanny in capturing the way I felt, and this song has stuck with me throughout my life since then. Because my dad was my biggest advocate, I've often wanted to tell him how much I love him "… in the living years." But this illness, with its dark and icy grip, had obscured my thoughts and feelings.

I was released after twelve days. Dr. Paul George, a psychiatrist at UVCH, wrote: "After being placed on Haldol and intermittently throughout the stay, she was quite rational. At that time she talked of her stressors being 'dating and relationships.' She became calm, cheerful, and friendly, indicating that she could not believe the things she had done prior to admission. She was discharged on Haldol and continued psychotherapy with Dr. Gibbons but stopped the medication shortly after discharge."

Faces Like Masks

*"Never limit yourself to the world; when the mind has no limits.
Do our eyes only see as far as the light will shine or shall we
discover our own sight when we allow our minds to discover the
wonders of God?"*

~Jill Campbell

In October of 1992 I was readmitted to the "lockdown" psychiatric unit. The medical record states, "The patient was acting bizarrely and having delusional thought disorder. She had been hospitalized in March of this year for a similar problem. She states she was put on Haldol and Zoloft, but as far as she knows, she quit taking the medication soon after she left the hospital. The patient is a normally nourished, normally developed, twenty-two-year-old white female. She stares unusually at things, and often states things that are completely irrelevant to what is being asked and to what we are talking about with the medical history. For example, she will say, 'The answer is Texas' without any reason to be saying 'Texas.'

"She does not appear to be in any acute physical distress. When approached, the patient was in the seclusion room with one-on-one supervision, lying on the bed. She did agree to come into the examining room for the interview. Her body movements were extremely erratic and generally without purpose. At one point she lay over backwards, resting the back of her head on the desk.

"She sat somewhat restlessly in the office chair, using signing and guttural speech intermittently and then occasionally asking, 'Can you hear, do you speak English?' and then talking clearly for a few phrases before reverting back to waving her arms and signing violently. When asked to speak English only and to put her hands in her lap, she did so for approximately ten seconds and then began banging her elbow very hard on the wall a number of times until asked to stop.

"She cooperated only marginally but was able to answer most questions, frequently winking, nodding her head, and whistling softly. Her hair was dangling and uncombed. She wore jeans and a T-shirt. Her moods changed quickly. She appeared to feign a cry for a few seconds. She said thereafter that she felt good. At another point she seemed more genuinely upset while commenting that she doesn't remember who she is. The patient behaved in such a bizarre manner that it is quite possible that there may be hallucinations. She spoke in disjointed phrases and sentences. These were not logical or goal-directed. At one point she looked at her hands, smiled and said, 'Aren't hands wonderful?'

"It was reported by the staff that the patient has seemed quite disoriented at times. Her impulse control is extremely poor and she has required one-on-one nursing care because of erratic and dangerous behavior. She has wandered in other patients' rooms and taken things off the walls. She broke a dish. She has been spitting at and on people. Her symptoms are essentially the same as on the first admission, at which time she was diagnosed as having brief, reactive psychosis, factitious disorder and mixed personality disorder with borderline obsessive compulsive and dependant traits. She has a concerned family and apparently a good premorbid level of functioning.

34

"The patient was restarted on Haldol and Cogentin, but the majority of the doses were refused by her. She was placed on the locked, secured unit, under one-on-one supervision. We will reinstitute antipsychotic medication. She will participate in individual, recreational therapy when appropriate. Discharge plan: If she can stabilize sufficiently, she may be able to remain in the area and continue her schooling. She apparently lives with her sister. Appropriate follow-up therapy will be arranged."

During this hospitalization I was again given a room with grated bars on the window. Windows seemed my only connection with the outside world.

> *Gazing through the window of my soul*
> *Riding the crests of the breasted clouds*
> *Gently grazing the lips of the whispering hills*
> *Speaking softly wind blows in my ear*
> *I hear. I nod back to reality.*

My bed was again in the center of the room, and I was given a sheet, pillow, and blanket to put on it. It was cold. I wasn't allowed to use the bathroom in isolation for fear that I would drown myself. It was locked. I had to urinate in the cup they gave me for water. As in my earlier hospital stay, the medication made me intensely thirsty. I fell often on the hard concrete floor, the walls in the room were padded but the floors were cold and solid like ice. The lights were blinding and I found sleep difficult. I can't remember if I had socks, I had no shoes. When I walked on the floor the iciness felt like hot coals and nails on my feet so I crawled on my hands and knees in the recreational room. My sensations were heightened; once again I was hallucinating.

> *Faces like masks*
> *Two sides to every man*
> *Unfamiliar faces ask who I am*

I ask them for water
Denied regularly at night
My eyes blinded by the light
My mouth drier than a desert
Nothing to quench my thirst

The "prisoners" and I devised signs of my own making to communicate through these grated windows. There was a courtyard in the center of the hospital with rooms and windows facing onto it. This was the window from which I viewed my life. After being locked up for a few days, I thought there was going to be a fire. The signals were my communication with others in my frenzy to execute the exodus. My mission to rescue my fellow inmates was complete. Everyone was safely released from their cell to escape the fire, but I was still locked in my prison.

Sometime later that week, I was released from isolation. Although it was supposed to protect me from myself, it would haunt me for years to come. The white walls, barred windows, white bedding and cement floor did nothing to lift my spirits. I felt completely isolated and it seemed only to exacerbate my loneliness. There was nowhere to escape to and I found the confinement further damaging to my soul. A few days later, I was allowed to walk around the inner court of the hospital. I met and talked with a man from the Navajo reservation. I gave him twenty dollars, and we talked for some time. I still remember his kindness. I'm not sure if he ever returned to the reservation, but I remember his pride in being an American Indian. I found myself wishing I were as kind as he. He reminded me of the following picture that I drew my senior year in high school.

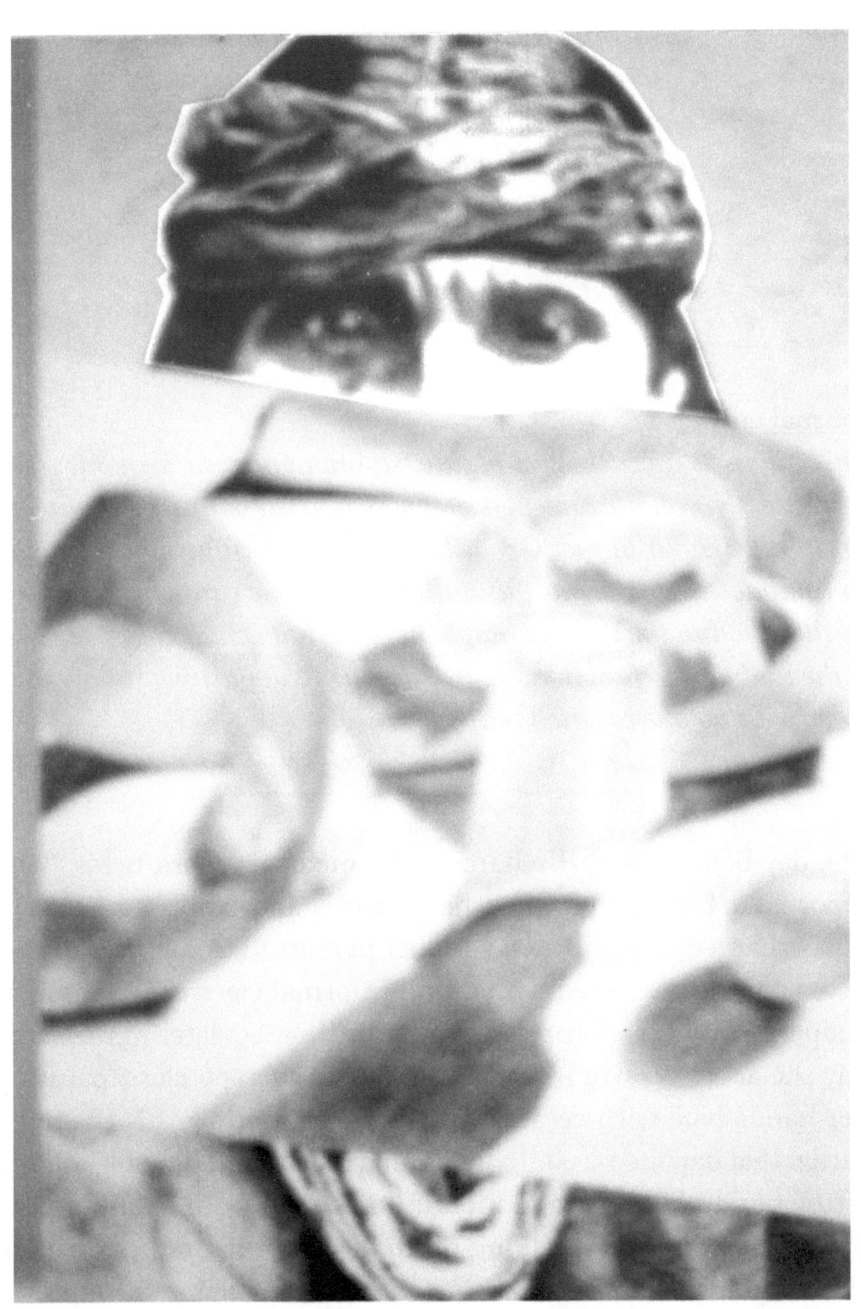

Jill Campbell (Ebony pencil)

Fortified memories hit the stone
Absorbing the echo hidden by the wind
Crumbling to the valley like dust
Echoes resounding against granite walls
Breaking down the granite face
Releasing the echo...
The stone can't hide in the wind
It trickles in your fingers
Into forms to be molded

Journal entry:
This illness is a cruel twist of fate, so impacting, so demonic, and so restlessly present and persistent. It is tireless in its attempt to drain all life out of me. Or is it the empty restfulness, the energy so compacted, or the painful dullness? Is it the exuberance for life pushing you to the unimaginable heights that are so coveted? Or is it the inability to function, so maddening real, pushing me over the edge, with no one to catch me?

~~~~~~~~~~~~~~~~~~~~~~~

The day before I was discharged, the medical record reads: "She reported to her therapist that she felt better and expressed a wish to be discharged and returned with her parents to Colorado. On this occasion, she presented with a smile, normal voice tone, pleasant, cooperative, with appropriate reality testing. Yet later in the same day she acted bizarre in her occupational therapy class, painting her hands blue with ceramic paint. When seen by this therapist earlier that day she was initially signing as if deaf and mute, holding a rose bud to her nose and mouth (to prevent from breathing the polluted air), but then talking normally about her father's fishing skills and her desire to go fishing with him."

I vividly remember the scent of that rose.

Before the onset of bipolar, I reached out to those in distress, such as DiDi, Elizabeth, and Bruce Douglas. I saw the good in people and it was natural for me to see the needs of others. I wanted to emulate Princess Diana, her beauty, kindness, and compassion. I was a beautiful person both inwardly and outwardly and I liked who I was. However, after the onset of the illness, I became self-consumed and sank into states of debility, depression, and mania; I walked a fine line between helping others and reaching out for the wrong reasons. Sometimes voices in my head led me down broken paths and the trail back was not easy to follow. On one occasion I followed a man with a beard and mustache to the pet store because I thought he was Jesus; when the man didn't wait for me I felt like Christ had forsaken me. Tears rolled down my face, as I felt that I was not worthy of His love.

I only saw in the mirror the nightmare I was living and my beauty, which had faded fast. It became impossible for me to remember the slender 150-pound accomplished soccer player and confident runner named Jill. The marathon I ran in St. George, Utah, in 1990 was not nearly as difficult as the marathon of my life. During manic phases my delusions led me to believe something I was not—a hero saving those in danger, an ambassador to the lost, Princess Diana. I now became the one who needed help and compassion from others, and at times I didn't even know I needed it.

The Nightmare Is Real

"Sometimes I wish I had cancer instead; mania eats at your soul until you feel like dying inside. Only you don't."

~Jill Campbell

My mom and dad drove over to Provo from Denver in October 1992 to rescue my broken spirit and to sign my release from the hospital. Although Kristin was adamant that I should stay at BYU, I was discharged into my parents care; outpatient therapy would be arranged in Colorado. During the return trip to Denver a few days later, I had a continual sensation that the highway was trembling and quaking. I still hadn't come down from my manic phase. My parents were advocates for my mental health. But this was new to all of us and extremely baffling. So many questions—why was this happening? Will it last forever? Why the religious overtones to everything? The doctors convinced them that it was the nature of the illness. We found out later that bipolar illness does take on religious overtones, even if you're not religious. We were all eager to find out what was wrong with me. We were scared and confused and we all needed some answers.

My bipolar diagnosis would forever impact the way I see life and how life sees me. I would be at home almost a year and a half. I spent large portions of my days at home lying on the couch. I couldn't keep awake and then I couldn't stay asleep. The days were torturous while I rested on the couch, and the nights were the same. They melted into one another, and life seemed endless and hopeless.

My mom was my best friend and helped me to see beauty around me when I could no longer see anything. I walked their expansive gardens with her to awaken my soul, while my father prepared meals to nurse my body. Dad helped me back to sanity with his love, as well as his wonderful gourmet cooking. After having experienced a phobia of food in the psychiatric hall, his meals never tasted so good. He was between jobs, which was providential; it meant that his only job was to look after me.

He went with me to see a psychiatrist, Dr. Barkley Clark. Dr. Clark is a gentle and kind man, and I placed my ultimate trust in him. His compassion seemed almost God-like, and my confidence in him was unwavering. Many nights, I called him when I was hallucinating or depressed. His kind words and medical advice, oftentimes in the middle of the night, calmed my worst fears. During the most difficult times, he would call me daily to inquire about my well-being. The care and concern was above and beyond what most people experience. My first meeting with Dr. Clark began a succession of many visits that would span the next eighteen years. My dad took scrupulous notes during these meetings in order to help me to obtain the best care possible. My memories of my dad are very fond.

You rescued my soul
At my lowest valley,
You nursed me back
To sanity and reality
Despite your frailties,
Your gentleness, kindness
I can never repay

You rescued my soul
In so many ways

While I continued to recover, Kristin found running to be her sanity amid the uncertainty in my world. She also held a part-time job as an editor and managed to graduate in the fall of 1992. My formal education would end in the spring of 1994, over five years after starting college. I failed numerous classes and had to retake many. I believe my professors passed me with at least a C in several courses because I was incapable at that time of finishing my coursework. It may have taken me several more years to finish. I thank God for their grace and mercy.

Kristin's cross-country team at BYU qualified for nationals. My mom and dad and I flew to Indiana, where they were held that year. One morning I awoke in our hotel to a torrential rainstorm at 5 a.m. As might be expected from this inexplicable illness, I immediately decided to go for a run. I found a nearby park filled with large sculptures and danced around them in the pouring rain as if they were dancing with me. There was a lot of trash in this park and in the stream that ran adjacent to the street so I picked up handfuls of muddy trash caught in the drain, all the while condemning those who littered.

I walked across the street to a fast-food restaurant and threw away my trash and then went back and collected more trash. I then continued my morning jog. As I ran past the hotel where my parents and I were staying, I jumped cracks caused by "earthquakes." I felt the earth tremble under my feet, and this caused me to run faster and faster to escape the earth tremors. I started doing sprints back and forth in front of the hotel. I fell in front of a gas station and the attendant came over and asked me if I was all right. I said I was fine and continued to run.

The color-coded patterns of the cars were directing me once more. Finally, drained of all my energy and exhausted, I fell into a water gate deep enough to drown. Somehow, my head rested on the jacket I had wrapped around my waist. I was found unconscious. An ambulance arrived at the scene, and the EMTs notified my parents; it was uncanny that they were able to locate them because a note from my dad on hotel paper was in my pocket. Upon returning to my room, I took a hot shower, put on the white robe my mother gave to me, and sat on the window sill. The headlights from the cars in the pouring rain were speaking to me, again.

The cross-country national championships were held later that day. As Kristin rounded the corner toward the finish line, I raced after her. I went at breakneck pace through the flags where the athletes were stretching and relaxing from the race. Kristin later would write: "The nationals proved to be a letdown when my parents brought Jill to Indiana for the last race of the season. My stomach, already nervous before the meet, had turned to absolute fright after the race, when I saw her run across the course aimlessly. God had not prepared me for this final race. I would finish near the end. Although disappointed, we managed to take tenth overall."

That evening my parents and I went to a barbecue restaurant. The place was full of tables packed together. Smoke billowed everywhere. Knives, forks, and spoons clattered from every direction. Loud laughter and talking permeated my every sense. My eyes watered, my ears vibrated, my mind awakened. I excused myself from the table to go to the restroom. The bathroom was filthy. I picked up all the dirty paper towels strewn across the floor. I couldn't bear to use the toilet. I came out and went directly outside crying, my mom followed me and I explained to her how I was feeling; the bathroom was disgusting even for a person who wasn't hallucinating; however, it seemed more exaggerated to me. Once again, the bipolar had heightened my senses. It seemed as though my last links with joy and reason were severed. On the return flight to Denver, Benadryl calmed the mania and my agitation. I returned home with my parents and welcomed visits with Dr. Clark. I found the sessions engaging and thought provoking.

So many days
You rescued my soul
From the uncertainty
Of it all
I felt your strength
Your wisdom endless

The feared diagnosis came during my senior year when I returned home. Dr. Clark presented what I had been experiencing over the past two weeks "...of suspiciousness, feeling bugs on her skin, and experiencing earth tremors while riding in the family car. Her symptoms progressed over ten days to include an agitated high energy state, hypersensitivity to sensations, racing and confused thoughts, and visual and auditory hallucinations."

A review of my past history revealed I had been experiencing symptoms of hypomania (a less severe form of mania) since approximately the age of fifteen. Dr. Clark concluded that I was "a very bright young woman who now hopes her illness is stable enough to allow her to finish her undergraduate studies at BYU. She has been a delight to work with."

While at home in the spring of 1993, I was asked to help coach the Overland High School girls' soccer team, the same program in which I had played just five years earlier. I admired my coach, Bruce Brown, because he had been influential and instrumental during my soccer career. I considered him a great friend and confidante. It was a struggle for me to coach at this time due to my overwhelming feelings of paranoia. I often felt that everyone knew what was wrong with me. I had little or no confidence in my ability to coach them and often found myself in tears. On one occasion Coach Brown left me on the field with the girls and they rallied around me, saying how much they enjoyed having me coach them. We traveled to Arizona for spring break but I felt isolated, and it was difficult for me to travel and feel a part of the program. Although I loved soccer, I would turn my back on coaching. My illness greatly lessened my passion for soccer and left me swirling downward into another cycle of paranoia and anxiety—and a deeper penetration into mania.

CHAPTER SIX:

A Companion in the Darkness

"What greater earthly good is there for two human souls, than to feel that they are joined for life?"

~George Eliot

Although my parents supported me with my schooling, they had reservations about my returning to school without a competent doctor in Provo. The effects of the medicine were still unstable at that time. A psychiatric update from Dr. Clark dated December 30, 1993, states that, "Ms. Gebhart has been under my care for bipolar mood disorder. Her mood had been stable for approximately two months from early October 1993 through early December 1993 while being maintained on Lithium, Carbamazepine, and Perphenazine. In mid-December, Ms. Gebhart began to experience a disturbing intensification of emotions about family members, followed within one week by the onset of more rapid thoughts, sleep disturbance, and an idea that she possessed the power to bring about world peace. These symptoms occurred within the context of her preparing to return to college at BYU for the first time in one and a half years.

"As of this date, Ms. Gebhart's thoughts have slowed, she is now sleeping well, and she has regained an accurate appraisal of her capabilities to affect the world. But as a result of this recurrence of symptoms, Ms. Gebhart is understandably more concerned about her ability to adjust to a return to college life away from home and the support of her family.

"My hope is that Ms. Gebhart's current episode of symptoms will remain quiescent on the current regime of medications, and that she will be able to complete a successful transition back to college life in Provo. Please let me know if there are questions or concerns."

It terrified my parents to have me so far away, and Dr. Clark suggested that I attend Colorado State University, where I would be closer to home. In my determination to finish my education at BYU, I returned to college in January of 1994. I was convinced that I was supposed to return to BYU.

While there, I met the man who would change my life.

I first met Dan at a dinner we had with several of our friends. I arrived late and everyone introduced themselves to me. He was over six feet tall, light brown hair and blue eyes. He was every girl's dream. He had served a two-year mission to Santiago, Chile, and was sensitive and kind. As soon as Dan introduced himself, I knew I was going to marry him.

I dreamed of you
Every passing day
One glance and I knew
You were the one to stay
Your whisper in my ear
Of love and tenderness to follow
I had longed to hear
After my heart was so hollow
My pleas to the Father
Only enhanced my desire

To meet a man
Built through the refiner's fire
That man was you
Someone with virtue and vision
Integrity followed you
A man with a mission

He didn't have the same conviction that I did at first; however, it would only be months before he asked me to marry him. I talked to him after dinner was over, and I knew this was the man I wanted for my husband. We talked about my love for Colorado, his desire to live there, his mission, and his master's program in accounting. On our first date, Dan and I spent hours talking and we stayed out long after closing time at a nearby hamburger joint. He sang to me and played the guitar. A wonderful romance began...dining in Salt Lake City...hours in the fine arts center where he played the piano for me...attending the ballet. A few of my most memorable dates include singing and playing the guitar together and riding scooters at night. We left notes on each others door every morning.

Eyes Dancing

The meaning of love unknown to me
But holding my hope of love near
You walked into my life unexpectedly
Laughing and loving away my fear

Eyes sparkling in the firelight
Smiling unknowingly of plans untold
Uncertain, my imagination took flight
Bursting with excitement, feeling bold

Our eyes entwined for a moment in time
Confused by my feelings my eyes danced away

Emotions intensely on an upward climb
Our souls touched saying what words cannot say

Eyes dancing to a faster beat
Controlling words as we let our souls speak
Again and again our eyes meet
Faster and faster eyes dancing, feeling weak

Two souls losing touch with reality
Soaring in a world of their own
Flying away to a higher locality
Together loving deeper than we had known

He speaking softly with sincerity
My spirit overwhelmed with trust
Canyon fire burning with clarity
Spilling my soul upon earth's dust

Stars reflect the beauty of his face
Rushing water gently singing
Wind through trees on a whispering chase
Visions of eternity ringing

Dan and I were married several months later in the San Diego temple on the 13th of August. It was truly the greatest day of my life. We made promises to one another to live our lives so we could be together for eternity. It was incredibly beautiful.

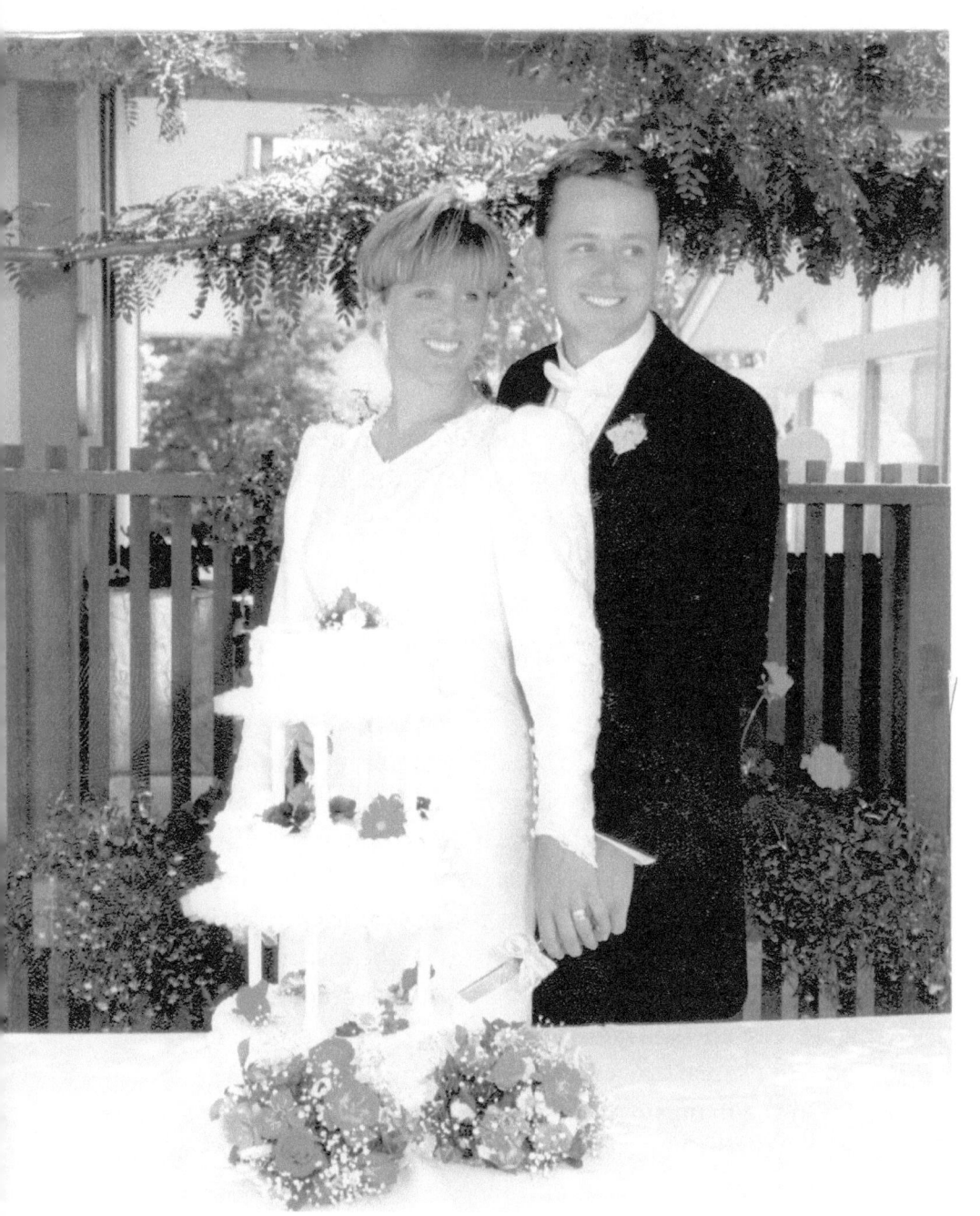

August 1994

Your love conquered my soul
My heart aching to be your wife
The plan that would make my life whole
Man to take woman, giving her life
Strengthened by my gentle prayer
With His hand He guides me
As man and wife burdens we share
On the path to eternal glory

Following the ceremony, we had a lovely reception in a room that overlooked the San Diego Bay area. We took pictures in front of the beautiful catamarans. At the reception, he played the piano and sang a song by Kenny Rogers, "Love the World Away." I stood next to the piano while he looked at me—we were completely in love. We would never have guessed the darkest windings that were ahead for us.

Kristin and Erik were married one week later in the Denver temple on the 20th of August.

Kristin, Erik, Dan and I had a beautiful double reception in Colorado at my parents' home. It was held in their unbelievably lovely back yard, with its large sweeping lawn and sloping hill. Surrounding the grassy area on all sides are flower beds rising in tiers with masses of blooming roses, irises, pansies, hibiscus, day lilies, and much more. Strawberries, rhubarb, green beans, and pea pods fill a flower bed on the west end of the lawn. Evergreens, a blue spruce, a maple, and an ash tree hover over the flowers on the north side of the grassy area, providing the blossoms relief from the summer heat. On the patio surrounding the hot tub, a locust tree shelters pansies, its roots bursting through the red brick. Tomato plants in wooden tubs surround the entrance to the house.

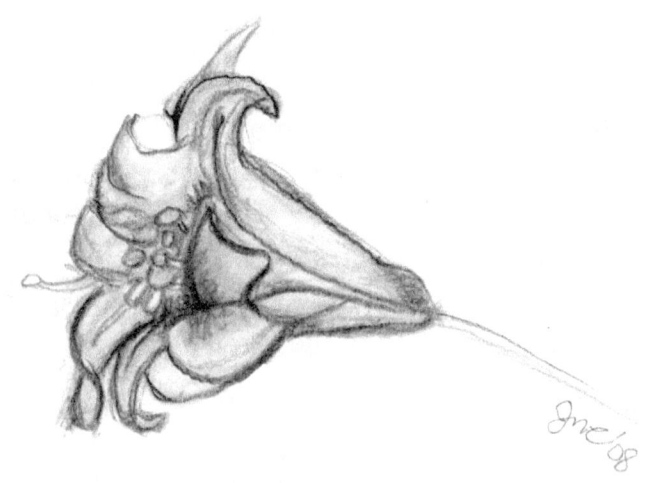

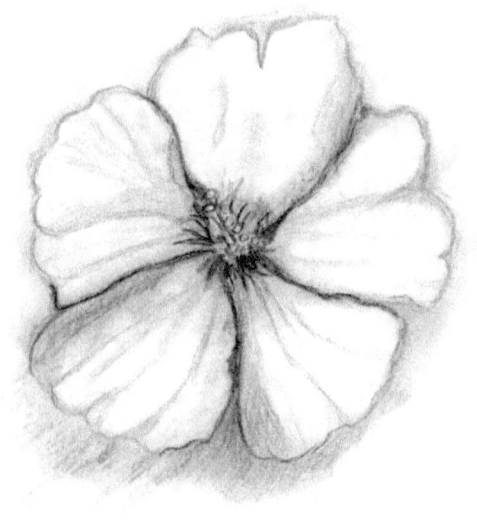

The hot tub was covered with royal blue and white linens with a beautiful awning. This would serve as a buffet table for finger foods and pasta salads. On the west side of the lawn a string quartet played music. At the center of the lawn an aisle runner was placed. With each of us on both sides of him, my Dad walked Kristin and me up the runner to the top of the hill where chairs were set up to witness the ring ceremony. Many of our parents' longtime friends and our own friends were present. Dan and Erik sang a song by Paul Simon titled "The Wedding Song," as Erik played the guitar. It was a splendid reception in the "Rose Garden."

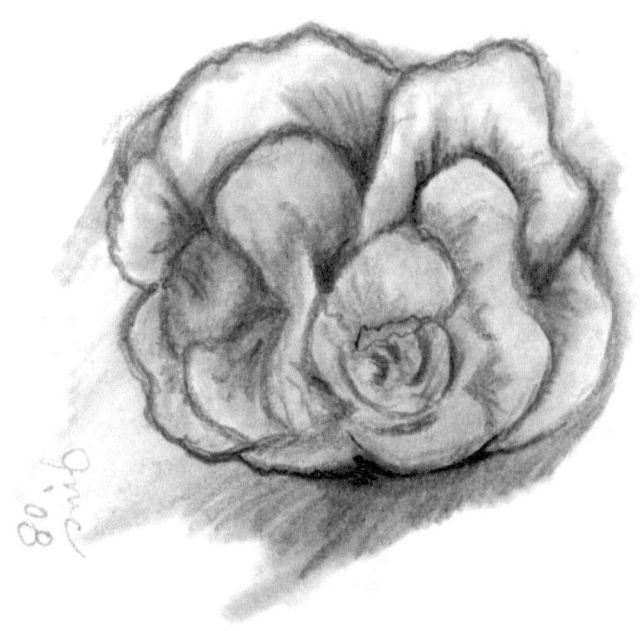

Fragrance, beauty, delicacy
The peace Rose dwells
As seasons change.
Flowers are a reminder
Of all that's good at home

Our honeymoon was a trip from California to Las Vegas to Steamboat Springs in Colorado. We played tennis, went hiking, rode the gondola up the mountain and biked down the ski slope that no longer had snow.

We returned to Provo in late August and spent the fall and winter semester in a small basement apartment on Cedar Avenue. It was dark, with no natural light, and it led to a new bout of depression. However, it was cozy and a memorable experience, and we shared good times together despite our poverty. Our halogen light would serve as a Christmas tree where we put lights up and twisted it around the standing light. Our only furniture was our bed, a papasan chair, and a small patio table in the kitchen that was adorned with a checkered white and blue tablecloth.

Rent was cheap, but neither of us were employed. I was just starting a job selling clothes at Layne Bryant (an upscale store for women's clothes in large sizes) on commission. I went to work trembling and shaking. I felt like it was the 1950s during the Red Scare. It seemed like everyone was watching me. This job lasted only a few days, because I experienced anxiety and paranoia. After I quit, I started job searching again; however, this time I thought I could do some beadwork at home so I wouldn't experience the anxiety and fear I was feeling about being around people. It consisted of making necklaces and was very intricate and paid very little, which contributed to my sense of low self-worth and no confidence to hold a decent job. This was the first stage of a long and strenuous trek that my husband would willingly and unknowingly travel with me.

Dan and I decided it would be best for me to go home and get professional help from Dr. Clark. We were separated for several months! Daily we conversed on the phone; the separation was painfully lonely. I missed Dan terribly. However, this change would prove helpful to my mental health. He joined me in April when his coursework at BYU was finished. We were expecting our first child in September.

CHAPTER SEVEN

A Gift From God

"There is no living in love without suffering."

~Thomas à Kempis

Children were born to us
God blessed us with one of each
He gave us a unique challenge
Only he knew our beseech

The miracles and blessings followed
As each one depended on us
Gratitude replaced hearts so hollow
And filled us with tenderness

During the summer of 1995, Kristin and I were each pregnant with our first child. We worked together at Holly's Soccer 2000, a soccer shop where she was the manager and I was her employee. We balanced books, sold shoes, and stocked shelves. We opened shop at ten, giving us time to walk and swim together before we went to work. We were in quite good shape considering we were seven months pregnant. Dan took courses at the University of Denver so we could be together. We would return to Provo the following year for a short visit when I graduated, six years after I began, with my bachelor of humanities and he with his master of accountancy. Dan obtained a position with Arthur Anderson, a grueling job that required him to stay up continuously for two nights and three days. He took his CPA exam and received his license. After Brandon's birth, we moved out of my parent's house and found a small townhome a couple of miles away.

Brandon Curtis Campbell was born prematurely in September, during a major snowstorm. In the howling blizzard many trees fell down. It was difficult to shovel out our car because of the huge drifts. My membrane ruptured but I wasn't having contractions, so they gave me Pitocin at the hospital to speed up the contractions. After he was born, we cried—he was so beautiful with sandy brown hair and deep blue eyes. We held him for a few minutes and then to our terror we saw he was turning blue.

Dan quickly rushed for a nurse. Brandon, as a preemie, was having trouble breathing, so they put him on oxygen. They did multiple tests on him to see if his heart was fine and transferred him to the neonatal intensive care unit at The Children's Hospital because his heart was not working efficiently. He was diagnosed with mitral-valve regurgitation; the mitral valve was deformed, and the blood was flowing backward into the left ventricle, enlarging the heart. The doctors didn't know what the next step would be. We were frightened by all of this but tried to keep our faith strong. Brandon had a tube inserted in his trachea and an NG tube inserted in his nose in order to feed him. He would stay at Children's Hospital for three months. We brought a music box with soothing music that we played in his "crib." Stuffed animals lined his bed, and his outcome looked positive. It was a thrilling moment when I was able to hold him, but how I yearned to have him in my arms without those tubes!

The steps toward Brandon's recovery were each steps of joy: months later when he was taken off the ventilator; the day I was allowed to feed him with a bottle for the first time; the first time he cried out loud. Dan and I spent many days at the hospital with Brandon. Dan missed school often; however, his professors were kind and understanding. Friends brought meals, even though we were at the hospital almost every minute of every day. We even stayed several nights in a makeshift cubicle with other parents in similar circumstances.

Just when we thought it was difficult having Brandon in the NICU, we realized others had it much, much worse. The couple staying in the cubicle next to us were in the hospital because their two-year-old daughter was brain dead. The dad had reversed the car in the driveway thinking everyone was clear from the car, and he ran over his daughter, who would live for only a short while. His wife was extremely supportive and a great comfort to him.

We tried to be positive despite the problems we feared Brandon might face in the long run. Life didn't seem as hard, and our spirits were good at this time. We had a lot of support from others and from our faith; both Dan's and my parents were a great support to us. We brought Brandon home just before Christmas. We had been staying with my parents for almost eight months and were grateful for their generosity.

My memory fails me and I can't remember what happened between 1995 and 1998, before Kayla was born, although I remember what a joy it was to raise our son, Brandon. It was an encouraging time because I experienced few significant mood changes for almost three years. Dr. Clark successfully managed my medication until I became pregnant again which changed my body chemistry and led to another onset of symptoms.

Journal entry:
Another happy day! Brandon smiled for the first time. He is a darling and a joy and he cried every time I set him down.

~~~~~~~~~~~~~~~~~~~~

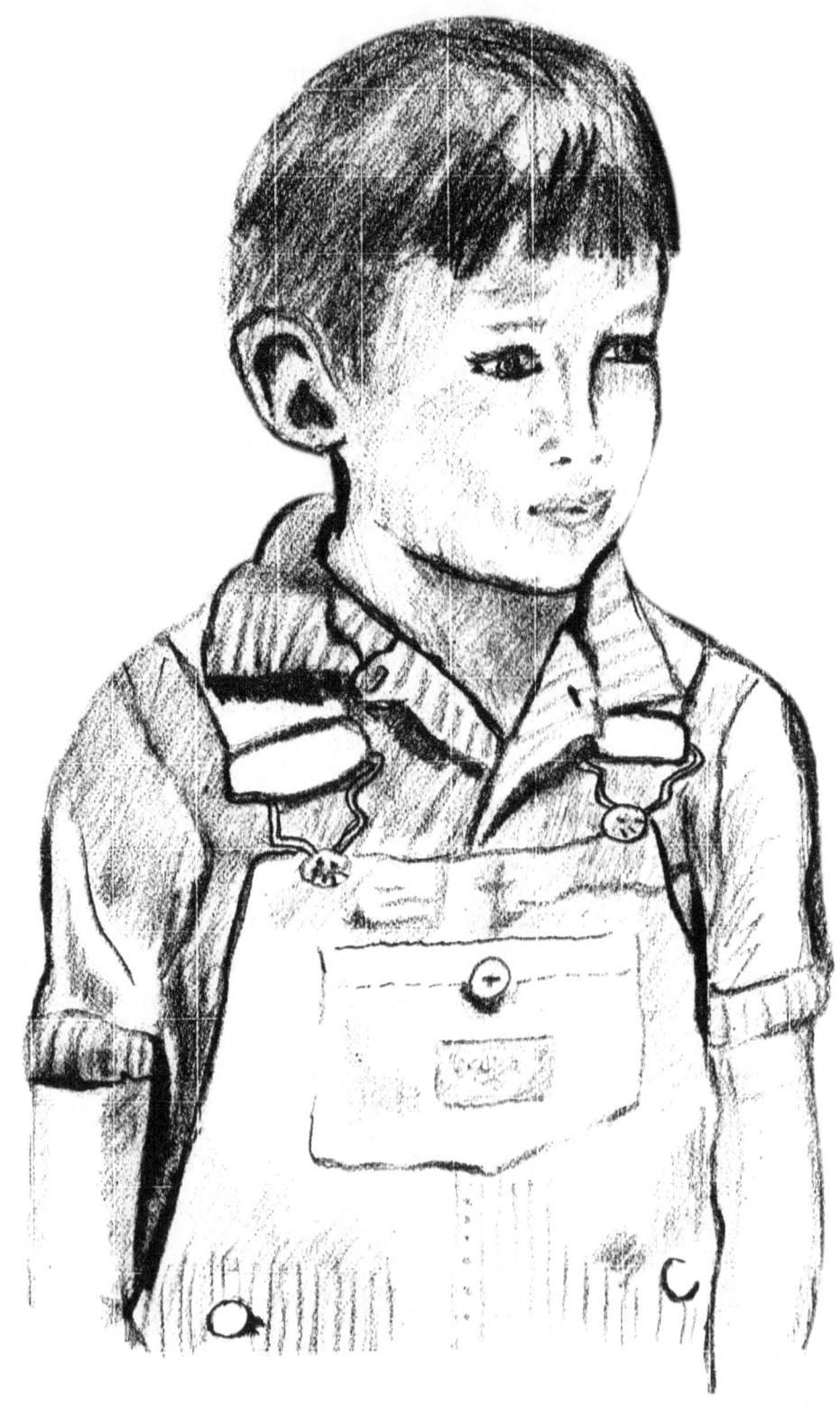

Brandon

I'd climb mountains for you
I'd sail the ocean blue
I'd forge valleys for you
I'd walk the world to be with you
You'd push me to the shore
So I could dive below
I'd drop from the sky
If only I could go where you go
I'd walk through deep forests
I'd run through fields of red
I'd walk on stormy seas
With clouds spinning over my head

During all that time my illness was lurking in its lair, cunningly biding its time. Then it slithered out unexpectedly. My next delusion took place when Dan was out of town. When Brandon was three and I was still pregnant with Kayla, we went to an appointment at The Children's Hospital. We were on Colfax Avenue upon returning from the hospital, in a location where poverty is prevalent. We stopped at a 7-Eleven to get something to eat. I was dressed in a black dress and pearls—I was hallucinating and thought I was Princess Diana.

As we were getting out of our car, I motioned a homeless man over to our car in order to give him money to get something to eat. I went over to where three other homeless men were sitting. One man said he was Andrew Jackson, the seventh president of the United States. From my perspective, we were all mentally ill. Although my son was cowering behind me, I wasn't nervous. A few kids drove their car through the alley on the west side of 7-Eleven. They told me not to be scared. I was far from scared, and we conversed for almost one hour. Although I know that these were merely troubled people like myself, today it gives me chills to think about the situation I put Brandon and myself into.

On another occasion I had Drew, Kristin's eldest son, and Brandon. I took them to the grocery store after 11 at night. When we finished shopping, one of the car seats wouldn't hook. Because I weighed over 230 pounds due to gestational diabetes, edema, toxemia, and Lithium, it was difficult to hook the car seat. I stopped at fire station #11 to see if they could help me and was irate at how long it took for someone to respond to the doorbell. Finally three firefighters came to help me. I swore at them. I'm not sure why they didn't arrest me for swearing and cursing at them. Mania had settled in and I couldn't escape it. Relentlessly it followed me everywhere I went, carving its own reality.

My world was distorted and life was painful. Food became my only source of comfort, and the combination of depression, medicine, and ill children pushed me to my highest weight of 285 pounds. I would eventually lose the weight over the next few years, but gained almost 100 pounds back. Later, I lost that as well. Life was painful, I lost everything I ever wanted and ever had. My life had changed dramatically. And the sorrow I felt was immense. These were dark days for me. Depression seeped into every facet of my life, and my confidence decreased as my anxiety increased. I could no longer see in front of me. I was not the person I had seen in the mirror a mere ten years ago. The laughing, beautiful, carefree person I used to be was no longer the person I saw.

My husband never failed me, even though I felt like I had failed myself. He always made me feel beautiful, and sometimes I almost believed it.

To the man I love:
I pray I haven't failed you
All I ever wanted was forever

For God has given me this path
Tears flow and then we laugh
You have walked the road
Hand in hand as life unfolds
Mysteries of my life
Like a double-edged knife
Walk with me, by my side
Accompany me on this night
My search for eternity
Became my serenity

Throughout most of my pregnancy with Kayla I was delusional and hardly realized that I was so overweight. My legs were the size of an elephant's, swollen and painful. I thought this was part of the "master plan." Although it took me several years to lose the final hundred pounds, my obsession with the scale would follow after losing most of the weight. I still struggle with it today. My fear of gaining weight is immense.

During my last months of pregnancy with Kayla, my body temperature soared. We had no air conditioning, and it was blistering hot at night. The plastic sheet I put on the bed would allow me relief as I poured cold water on the bed and all over my body. This helped but only briefly. I was agitated and restless, and sleep eluded me. During the daytime, I would soak my cotton maternity shirt in cold water. When my shirt would dry, I would soak it again. Elton John's tribute song to Princess Diana, "Candle in the Wind," soothed my distraught mind and body as I took long ice-cold baths in the middle of the night. I did this over and over—I believed I was Princess Diana. If only I were so regal and so kind. I'm not sure Dan ever rested well, but I thought I fooled him as to my true state of mind. My reflection in the mirror was distorted, and I couldn't see the real me. Perhaps this was a blessing.

Music fills her soul
Alone, one woman longs to feel whole

Although it may seem as if I experienced mania and depression continuously, I actually had long periods of remission where I neither experienced a significant change in mood or hospitalization. Despite these ongoing challenges there were good times.

Journal entry:
Brandon memorized 'Twas the Night Before Christmas at the age of three. This was a golden year for us. Christmas was normal—no hospitalizations for any of us! Brandon continues to amaze us and is a joy. Dan is my best friend and has tolerated more than any person can imagine. "For God must know, I love you so." (Barbara Streisand)

Brandon was writing a sentence on the computer and he put exclamation points at the end. He said, "Mom look, excitement marks." He was doing multiplications and I asked him if he was doing homework, and he said "No, I'm doing this for fun"—and he was serious! He is an absolute delight, although at times he is willful. A good trait. We have to rush him in the morning to get ready; he is so full of thoughts that we can't keep him focused.

He loves math, music, hockey, and baseball. He is an exceptional piano player. He is an absolute delight.

We haven't had television for over two years, and it has changed our lives. I'm not always sure what is going on, but I'm also not burdened, depressed, or obsessed about world issues.

My Darling

"My tears of yesterday are sorrow, and my tears rain today, happiness for the morrow, cannot compare to this day."

~Jill Campbell

Kayla was also born prematurely on October 12, 1998. She had many health problems over the next few years that we were not prepared for. Prior to her birth, I was admitted to the hospital to be treated for edema, gestational diabetes, and toxemia, as well as mania. Because I was experiencing mania, they confined me to a maternity ward instead of transferring me to a psychiatric hospital. It would have been too much of a risk for Kayla and me. Our heart rates were soaring, so they had to perform an emergency C-section.

Everything happened so fast, but I remember Dan at my side, which reassured me greatly. I was barely coherent and never heard Kayla cry, because she never did. It took several minutes before she started to cry, and it would be hours before I saw her in the NICU. When I saw Kayla for the first time, she was hooked up to IV fluid and had tubes in her throat and in her nose. Her face was puffy and she was barely recognizable as a human newborn.

Both of my babies' hospitalizations were similar, and the first time I saw Kayla my memories of Brandon's stay at The Children's Hospital flooded my mind and caused me great anguish. The three months that Brandon spent in the hospital hooked up to tubes seemed easy compared to the ten month stay that Kayla had at TCH. This was a devastating time, and my disease fed on the misery. We put Brandon in daycare because I was in no condition to take care of him. With Kayla's hospitalization, I was alone with my dark thoughts and feelings. This would prove harder to deal with than I ever imagined. I felt hopeless.

> *Dissonance in my heart*
> *My mind tearing me apart*
> *Discordance in my soul*
> *Aching to be whole*
> *Yesterday stealing a piece of tomorrow*
> *As I linger in my sorrow*
> *Building dreams in the corners of my mind*
> *Wondering how my life will be defined*
> *Diverging paths grasping my hand*
> *Uncertain, I roam this desolate land*

Kayla, like Brandon, was diagnosed with mitral valve regurgitation, which means that the valve between the left ventricle and the right atrium was defective. It would leak blood back out the valve and into the ventricle. Kayla also had myocardial spongiosum, where the left ventricle is spongelike; the valve defect and spongy muscle enlarged her heart, as well as her ribcage. The doctors believed that both Dan and I are carriers for this type of heart condition and that it was not due to my medication. As a preemie, she also suffered from tracheomalacia. Her main airway wouldn't stay open when she breathed, but miraculously her cartilage grew back and held her airway open. Neither one of them have suffered any long-term effects from these heart conditions.

One week after my emergency C-section, I walked more than ten miles to Safeway in order to cast my vote on election day, a needless trip that presented itself to me as totally logical and reasonable. I found a seat at the volunteer table while I studied the issues and was so intent that I failed to notice Channel 9 news. They asked me if they could film me; fortunately, I declined what could have been a possibly embarrassing live interview. I called Dan to tell him that I walked to cast my vote; he told me to go home, but he didn't realize what a difficult task this would be for me.

I walked to a nearby Italian restaurant for lunch. I saw some missionaries from our church eating lunch and asked them if I could get a ride home; however, for insurance reasons they weren't allowed to give anyone a ride. They didn't know how desperate my situation was, and exhausted and in tears, I walked the opposite direction home in a loop. After several miles I found my way to a friend's house, and he gave me a ride home. In this manic state, the most illogical and fantastic ideas seem real and normal. Thoughts fly quickly and kaleidoscopic patterns emerge in the most unexpected places, keeping one engaged in the misconception. Then comes the downhill spiral.

In April of 1999, after Kayla came home from the hospital for a short time, I was severely depressed. The routine for her care was laborious and time-consuming, and life was complicated by my persistent and perplexing illness. Kayla was fed several times a day, as well as continuously at night, by a gastrointestinal tube—a buttonlike tube inserted in her stomach and connected to a 60 ml feeding syringe positioned above her head—while the formula dripped into her stomach. This procedure took thirty minutes or more four times a day, and she gagged every time I fed her because her esophagus was tied to keep her from throwing up.

This was heartbreaking to watch because there was nothing more we could do. The goal was to enable her to gain weight by keeping her from throwing up. Although she gained weight, she had to endure this uncomfortable procedure for three years. She would also be fed on a continuous pump all night long to gain weight. She received four medications four times a day around the clock through her G-tube. During my darkest times, my mom would call me every four hours to remind me that she needed her medicine and that she needed to be fed. In December, she came home on oxygen, and the huge oxygen tank served as a Christmas tree.

In April, during one of her short visits at home, I took Kayla to see her primary-care physician, who told me this was one of the worst cases he had ever seen. I was already depressed and this was the final, dreadful, blow. On the way home the thought of suicide entered my mind. I was a few blocks away from the hospital when I decided to crash my car into a 4x4 Ram construction truck. That would end the pain for both of us. I was going no more than twenty-five miles an hour; if I had been truly serious about it I might have gone faster.

The ambulance came, and the EMTs asked me if I was hurt; I wanted to scream "I'm spiritually dead." I told them I had tried to kill myself because the pressure of taking care of Kayla was immense and suicide seemed the only way out. It was an incredible blessing that Kayla and I were unharmed. My husband came to the ER room after the accident. With compassion, Dan just smiled at me and asked, "Jill, what did you do?" and gave another smile of reassurance. I was screaming inside and he knew my actions were a plea for help. I felt like I was failing everyone, especially our daughter.

I spent the entire day in the emergency room with a guard at my door and was then transferred to University Psychiatric Hospital by ambulance. This was a vacation, relieving me of the intense responsibility of caring for Kayla, a weight that was too shattering for my fragile state of mind. My mom took Kayla home with her because Dan needed to return to work. The next ten hours in the emergency room waiting for an ambulance to take me to the psychiatric hospital seemed like an eternity. While at University North Pavilion Hospital, I spent my time eating, sleeping, and neglecting myself. I felt horribly guilty for failing my daughter, for not being able to handle the reality and extreme difficulty of her illness. I desperately needed help. Depression took up its destructive residence in me, only this time it was caused both by my illness and my circumstances—and no amount of medicine could cure it.

Kayla was hospitalized off and on over the course of ten months. Dan's parents, Lori and Ken, travel by motor home all over the country; however, they traveled to Colorado in order to help us during this trying time. They took turns taking me to the hospital every day, sometimes twice a day. I could no longer drive myself. I was depressed because Kayla was ill, and my guilt was overwhelming because caring for her seemed an impossibility. Many days I inwardly protested going to the hospital. I was so drugged that I often fell asleep holding Kayla. Lori stayed awake so Kayla wouldn't fall out of my arms. It's hard to believe now, but I resented this child who I could not care for. I have a poor recollection of those days due to my painful state of mind and the medication I was given.

While she was in the hospital the doctors prescribed a continuous positive airway pressure, called CPAP. It seldom worked, and the alarms went off constantly. They decided that she would go home with it in an attempt to keep her airway open. Since it took great effort for her to open it once it closed, she expended more calories than she took in, thus making weight gain even more difficult. I stayed at the hospital overnight to see if I could handle the machine at home, but I was so drugged that I never woke up when the alarms sounded. The nurses adjusted the prongs over ten times that night. I was flabbergasted that they were going to send me home with this impossible contraption. The prongs were larger than the opening in her nostrils, uncomfortable for her and requiring constant adjustments from us. In order to hold the prongs in her nose, the tubes had to be attached to her head. Each time she moved, the tubes would be dislodged from her nostrils and the alarm would beep. She had to be completely asleep in order for the prongs to stay in her nose. They actually sent us home with this ridiculous machine.

Dan was temporarily working overseas, so the responsibilities for Kayla's health weighed heavy on my shoulders. I attempted to do my best operating a huge machine that was essential to Kayla's lung functioning but which didn't work properly. At eleven o'clock one night I was so exhausted that I admitted defeat and called the Visiting Nurses Association. They arrived and we devised a hat to hold the prongs in but this failed, too. The CPAP simply didn't work. The nurses had to leave, and I was left alone in this situation at 12:30 in the morning. I called Apria, the oxygen company, and was put on hold for over an hour, after which they said that there was nothing they could do without a physician's authorization. I stayed awake all night, exhausted and completely dejected. I laid down to sleep, but my concern for Kayla's health kept me awake. Kristin stayed with me that night, and she and Brandon slept in our bedroom.

During a medical conference held for Kayla the next day, the hospital personnel acknowledged the ridiculous expectation and responsibility they had given me—even for a healthy mother it would have been extremely difficult. We discussed the possibility of putting a tracheotomy in Kayla's airway, but after careful consideration Dr. Anne Halbaur suggested that we try the "iron lung," a breathing machine they used during the polio epidemic to keep patients alive. Kayla would use it at night and during naps. This finally proved helpful as it worked as a negative pressure ventilator to inflate her chest and made breathing much easier for her.

Each night that I slept in Kayla's room was challenging. Sleep was virtually impossible because the oximeter would go off intermittently and the iron lung took deep breaths regularly. This added to the maelstrom of my state of mind. Kayla's health was the most important thing and I felt like an around-the-clock nurse.

Journal entry:
Kayla, I want so badly to feed you and comfort you. I love you so much that I have to turn off my emotions sometimes, because the pain is unbearable. I don't want to hook you up to a machine, I want to watch you crawl and play and grow.

~~~~~~~~~~~~~~~~~~~

As it turned out, the iron lung proved highly beneficial for Kayla.

Agonizing over your every breath
Over your tiny soul so divine
Praying life would prevail over death
Not Knowing God's time

I lost you more each day
As fear lingered in my heart
Wondering if you were here to stay
As God acted out His part

It was His will for you to live
You fighting so valiantly
Your Life was His to give
To you He gave more abundantly

My tears of yesterday are sorrow
And my tears rain today
Happiness for the morrow
Cannot compare to this day

Praying over your tiny body
My dreams of you almost passed me by
I thought God would make you His
Never questioning why

Now I hold you in my arms
The gift I never can repay
Tears freely flow with gratitude
For my Father and His Son each day

The meetings with all the doctors, nurses, caseworkers, and respiratory therapists completely overwhelmed every part of me. Dan was an advocate for me when I had little or no capability. We talked openly about my mental illness, and to my relief, my suicide attempt was never mentioned. We discussed putting Kayla in foster care until I felt better; I could hardly believe I was considering giving my child up to another home, even temporarily. In my wildest dreams I never would have guessed I would be in a position where I would be forced to give up my child. It was heartbreaking.

The caseworker came to our house, and I filled out the paperwork. I felt dispirited and desolate that my child would be in a stranger's care. I was screaming inside. I rejected the foster care plan. The core issue became whether or not I could sleep during the night. Because sleep was crucial to my mental health, it was extremely important that I rest well. If Kayla could sleep all night in the iron lung, then I could take care of her. There was no debating the fact and I said that I could do it...not knowing if I really could— although as it turns out, I did!

I often took Kayla shopping; I rigged her stroller so the pump was attached to it, which meant I could feed her on a timed pump while I did my shopping. Her oxygen tank fit well in the basket of her stroller. I would put the entire stroller, pump, and oxygen tank in the oversized shopping cart at Costco. It was imperative for both of us that we get out and try to resume as normal a life as possible.

In January of 2002, the doctors removed her G-tube and we sent the "iron lung" back to the hospital. We were elated, and there seemed at last to be a light at the end of the dark tunnel. The tube had been a time-consuming process as I calculated and charted the calories she was taking in from table food and balanced it with the formula that she was being fed through her tube. During this time, Kayla was learning how to eat and to drink from a cup. I used a 5 ml syringe full of apple juice to get her used to the taste of food. At first she was full from being fed all night long on the pump, so when I tried to feed her she wasn't hungry. However, cutting back on the calories she took in through her G-tube enabled her to feel hungry and made it possible for her to eat table food. Velveeta cheese, guacamole, and pureed beef served as high-calorie foods—one teaspoon at a time. It was over six months before we could get her off her bolus feeds and feed her orally. Our efforts paid off, and she was soon eating everything.

At one time their health was delicate, and the worry consumed us. The fear of losing both of them was a constant reminder of how very fragile life really is for all of us. We never know when our time is up. The Lord has given us extra time with these two souls; they are truly gifts from Him. Every day when we kneel in prayer as a family we are grateful for the good health our children enjoy, as well as my health. We have been tremendously blessed.

Despite all her health problems, Kayla was still a typical three-year-old. She got into the Crisco vegetable shortening and smeared it all over the floor, her pajamas, and her face. Two days later, she took red permanent marker to the blinds. She also called 911, and the fire department called back to see if everything was OK.

Journal entry:

Kayla, at three and a half, is speaking remarkably well. She can count to twenty, skipping four and pronouncing twenty as "twenteen." When she walks, her loose curls bob up and down. Her eyes are large, blue, and the shape of almonds. She is very assertive and inquisitive. Kayla is enamored by her older brother. He plays with her all the time and makes her go into fits of laughter with his animation.

My Hidden Tears

"He found me in a long, unending night, in a lonely wilderness."

~Gloria Reed

November 1, 1999

Dear Dr. Clark,

The wisest, brightest, and most compassionate people are springing up at this moment in history. We think to ourselves, "There can be no cure for this disease at this time—it is too soon, too fast." But the truth of the matter is wisdom is at the center of science. Wise men and women are tapping into a power greater than themselves—called inspiration. Many new advances in technological science are shedding new light and breath upon the capacity to solve man's most troubling questions. Can I forgo my education, put it behind me, say it never was? No, I cannot. Why? Because my education spoke to me from the men and women throughout the centuries, as they discovered universal truths.

William Faulkner stirs my soul and speaks to me as if he had a conviction of life and death. He wrote, "I believe that man will not merely endure; he will prevail. He is immortal, not because he alone among the creatures has an inexhaustible voice, but because he has a soul, a spirit capable of kindness and compassion." Many of my friends were born centuries before I was born. Perhaps many of my friends will die, and their lives will continue long after I lay my soul to rest. Shall we say William Faulkner was not my friend, largely because we never walked the same pages of history? Faulkner spoke to me and I listened. His wisdom and love paved the way for a brighter future. Are we men and women prone to make the same mistakes? Certainly we are; but we are also creatures remarkably in tune with our divine potential—that potential giving way to the epicenter of wisdom.

During the earlier centuries men recorded their thoughts through journals, poetry, music, letters, art, and much more. It took weeks, months, even years to convey what they thought was so intensely vital to their expression and meaning in life. Centuries later, with a mere touch of one single button, letters, thoughts, wisdom, art, and knowledge are transmitted back and forth.

And you ask, "Why do I think I am entitled to believe a cure for my illness will be found?" There is no greater era than the era you, my friend, walk with me, through this journey in which you, through your industry and God-given abilities, have pursued a lifetime study to save men and women whose minds are missing the complex wires and chemicals to secure their ability to function. Confusing, perplexing, frustrating—utterly beyond my control. Therefore, I am completely holding your hand as you lead the way. Please don't let go—press forward. It is a living nightmare. The only blessing of this disease, at this time, is my lack of memory. I am thankful you have the technology and wisdom to forge ahead in uncharted territory. Now is the time—I will not let my life be in vain. Therefore my every step will be a concerted effort to alleviate the pain, sorrow, and suffering—not only for myself but for countless others who are affected by this dusting of Hell's flakes.

Your laughter embodies love, God given are your talents above. My eagerness to converse for a solution to reverse this hell. My godlike love for you has only been for a few. In the darkness of the night you've chased away my fears and softened my tears. You've given me my life back more abundantly. I cry tears of yesterday, but my trust in you is of today.

Dr. Clark,

I appreciate all you've done for me. But now I'm going to make bold on our friendship and ask for even more—I have some ideas, some of which I'm not sure I can express adequately. Please be patient with me. I no longer care about the requisition of my life as I once knew it, on an individual level. I'm concerned about our children, communities, and the quality of life as manifested by both of these. And perhaps this category does loom larger on a scale I have failed to mention—perhaps the illustration of Aaron and Moses applies in this case. My weary soul needs the strength of a man wise in such matters.

I feel as if I've been thrown off a vessel in the sea. The high tides, the ebb and flow of the sea, make it very difficult to keep my head above the water. But as the waves crest, I too ride to the top. I have several choices. I can continue riding the waves up and down, up and down, with a false hope that soon these ups and downs will take me to a better place, just enjoying the ride, but never approaching a safer place. A boat passes during the daylight, but I prefer to bob up and down. Twenty-four hours pass, and another day is on the horizon. Today is a new day; even though I've been treading water for twenty-four hours, I'm going to yell at the captain of the ship, maybe even thrash about in an effort to demand attention and possibly secure my safety.

And then another day passes, the sun sets, and with it the likelihood of spending another night alone, in the dark, with the realities of what darkness brings—sleepless nights that not even music can soothe. Sounds so penetrating that I jump at the sound of my own breathing. Sights so implacably confusing. Smells so intense I wish I could transform myself. Connections in the brain that allow you to trust the most distrustful, and distrust those whom are the most worthy of your trust.

In an attempt to find moments of lucidity and secure my thoughts of sanity, I choose not to acknowledge the magnitude that real spiritual influences have had on my healing process for close to two decades. The incredible underpinning that drives the mania results in a constant struggle to distinguish the true spiritual aspects of my life from the spiritual mania: what really is spiritual and what is delusional. The spiritual realm can be a constant guiding force as the greater of the two evils, mania and depression, takes shape—alternating one by one, in a vacillating vat of total confusion and absolute exhaustion.

These are the three states of being I experience: apathetic exhaustion, contented reality, and complete delusion. The totality of my being is not circumscribed in these three components but rather is explained as a reality by dissecting the parts that make me whole—whether good or evil. I often ask myself why a woman—once intelligent, beautiful, interesting, funny, kind, compassionate, successful, and goal-oriented—now finds herself subject to losing her soul, her animation, her body. Everything that she once held dear. Life seemed so perfectly beautiful, I thoroughly enjoyed visiting God's creation: to run with the sun as it rose over the mountains in the early light, to ride the dusty trail, to ski on the virgin snow, and to bike through streams as I gloried in the cold, wet water's tender touch.

Thankful am I for you—yes. Thankful for your love—yes. Thankful for your wisdom—yes. Thankful for the medications—debatable. I've lost my soul, my being, everything that makes me who I am.

You have fought with me
Ever so valiantly
My freedom comes at a cost
Yet I'm so lost

Sucked into this abyss
Darkened by light
Where is this bliss
Tortured by sight

Deafened by sound
A state of confusion
So very profound
A hauntingly real delusion

Lost in a dream
Yet so very real
I could scream
Life is so surreal

My ambitions in life are now being realized in ways my mind never explored. More than ever, I realize my love, my passion—in life and for life. My interest in the highest form of human life, you and me, is my study, my love, my adventure—one I eagerly embark on: to find the deepest, most intriguing manifestations of humanity. My connections to the human race are more divine and compassionately perfect. This journey is not one where I tremble and quake as I discover my individual capacity to triumph…or fail. No, I do not fear that. What I do fear is Life. I ask myself: Is my soul living up to its potential, am I quitting on the human race, are my problems more worthy of solving than my veteran friend who cries for compassion each day on the side of the road? My son and nephew beg me to find something that this man can have to eat. Each time I travel that road and, in my human frailty, forget that there is a man traveling a road without a soul, with an empty stomach, perhaps with a mind as fragile as my own, my soul cries out to this man, who may have been me.

Every day my heart swells up
Thinking of days gone by
Have I missed the better part
Or am I beginning to fly?

My tears are hidden within
I feel them rising to my head
I want to let them out
But my mind feels dead

Perhaps one fault of my illness is my inability yet eagerness to meet every soul that has placed his footstep on earth throughout the history of the world...and read every book that was ever written... listen to every song that has been sung...and hear the words of every child's inquiring questions. Is it manic to believe I can change the world? My way of changing the world is similar to those who have gone before me. Countless books have been, are being, and will be written. Knowledge passed down. Sanctified and glorified, as centuries of men and women have contributed strokes of genius, inspiration, and experience. Have you inquired of my school of study? If so, perhaps you'll understand. I love poetry, art, science, and literature. Yes, I, like you, have engrossed my mind in the pursuit of knowledge. Perhaps mine was fleeting and yours beautifully temporarily permanent.

Perhaps my only choice tonight will be to sleep on a bed of water—and pray that the pillow will be ice.

I'm still waiting to be rescued.

CHAPTER TEN

Soaring to Heights

"The springs of my life fell low, the shuddering of an unutterable dread crept over me from head to foot."

~Wilkie Collins, The Woman in White

During these difficult years, many different medications and combinations were tried, in various dosages. It took awhile to find the ones that protected me from this nightmare and didn't have crippling side effects. When Dr. Clark and I found the right combination I enjoyed a blessed reprieve for four years. After that period I was to experience one more drastic turmoil before reaching a peaceful shore.

The following hallucination occurred over a period of several weeks. Certain signals once again became my master map. I followed the cues when I saw one person drinking a bottle of water, color patterns of cars, cracked windows, or Gatorade bottles. I'd look for my next "cue" and then the next one. These signs would take me on long extended drives or walks. On one occasion I walked ten or more miles to fulfill my "mission." In some inexplicable way these missions were vitally important and were tied into world peace and harmony. I recorded my thoughts and the cues during this time:

Journal entry:
I had a dream, a vision. It was real. God gave gifts man to man... gifts of charity...given over time...would it be cyclical, creating a

domino effect contagiously spreading joy...Gatorade...water bottles...
cracked windows...three taps...dancing fingers...sign language...
people looking up heavenward...clasping hands...colors...wiping
mouths...drinking water...prove yourself Christian...the time is
near...togetherness...unity...one in Christ.

~~~~~~~~~~~~~~~~~~~~~~~

What I found in mania is a never-ending series of connections that demanded their completion according to the signals. The "plan" had to be carried out flawlessly. When a reaction or interruption was made contrary to the cues, the psychotic thoughts justified the alternation, and the connections continued at a rapid pace. I've traveled to a place most have never ventured.

There is a perplexing underlying facet that drives the confusion between reality, unreality, and spirituality—a constant guiding force as the two malevolent forces, depression and mania, take shape. They carry you on a seesaw ride of distortion and, eventually, absolute exhaustion. The distortion created an adventure not of my choosing, which I nevertheless had to embark on. The alternating communication between two evils became a raging battle in my mind. My interest was in both the deepest, darkest, and in the highest, most noble manifestations of humanity. That was where my journey always began, my adventure, my excitement to find the most profound and most intriguing realms of human life. I felt as if my wonder and imagination took flight, I thought about the trails I paved, the insights I gained, mountains I've climbed, sunsets seen through childlike eyes, the moon seen in the morning light. Beauty speaks so eloquently to my soul. While in this state, the strength I gathered from exploring humanity became a reservoir from which I drew living water to nourish and quench my thirst for knowledge, sought not within the barriers put in place to keep me in check, but expansive structures to climb as I continued my quest for learning.

Soaring to heights unimaginable. Seeing things only my eye can see. Distortions rack my brain with constant torment. My mind perceives it, and I believe it. Week after week, I suffer this excruciating pain. My mind clenched like a fist, my heart tied in a massive knot. How I ache to be whole. My mind takes me places I never wanted to go. Then exhaustion overcomes me; yet my brain, my mind, the intricacies of connections, are racing, racing at an unpardonable speed. Slowing them down is an impossibility. Locked in this chamber, I feel the distortions moving in and out, the walls moving in and out. What is reality?

~~~~~~~~~~~~~~~~~~~~~~~~~~~~~

Shapes draw me in
Lines hold me
Eyes feel the curves
Of the rolling hills
Touching the supple
Leaves far away
Eyes know the rough
Soil holding
Earth intact
Nevertheless
Eyes move from
Shadow to reality
Long enough to feel
Shadow moving in
Closer, distorting
Vision of the Earth

Journal entry:
I welcome the inviting activity that mania brings, I feel a greater sense of self-importance and imagination. I have the answer to world

peace, but it is shattered after the mania recedes. The reverie exits, and the dreadful depression and guilt enter. I believe so deeply in my perfected plan for universal harmony; but after the free fall, I bump into the wall of reality, the reality of what is wrong with me. Who will deliver me from these frightening, destructive upheavals? Once again I feel the walls closing in on me, and I can barely breathe.

Dreams of world peace fading away, my need for perfection—a goal that eludes me. My goal to meet Christ. But so unlike him, I am. I dream, I dream. But somewhere amongst the thistles and thorns, I am ensnared and snagged.

I believe that this delusion has been the most massive in scale.

~~~~~~~~~~~~~~~~~~~~~~~~~~~

My husband didn't know the complete extent of my mania. I called Dr. Clark several nights in a row, once at 2 a.m. He was a great source of comfort to me in this time of trial. I can't imagine living this nightmare without him.

In late December, I was admitted to Porter's psychiatric ward for depression, where I would spend Christmas day on the unit, as well as the next six days, mostly alternating between two states of mind. In my hallucinations, voices were telling me to kill myself. This was the bottom of the pit. I seemed to exist in an icy stillness of perpetual suspense. My memory blanks out most of it because the Clozapine I was given impaired my cognitive abilities. This last hospitalization was eleven years after the first one.

Dr. Clark wrote in his note for my admittance into Porter Hospital's psychiatric unit: "Since late October 2003, Ms. Campbell has struggled with rather continuous racing thoughts, shifting mood states, interrupted sleep, and misperceptions that strangers in the community are signaling her about religious decisions with world implications. Ms. Campbell and her family are exhausted and demoralized with the ravages of the current manic episode. We have been discussing the option of hospitalization to ensure her safety, to calm her current agitation, and to begin the next therapeutic option to try to stabilize her manic state."

Journal entry:
My tears rain a million drops for the sorrow I feel. The hallucinations hauntingly real. The fall ever so bitter, as the dark sky releases its tears. He took my dream away. How could I want more? How could I dream so intense when the father of lies exercised his pretense? I've fought to make my dreams real. Perhaps God's will shall prevail.

From the window of Porter psychiatric unit:

Moon hidden behind
The frigidity of
The winter freeze
And the silent trees

He speaks to me
From within the night
Golden, yellowy
Black by the twilight

Fir branches break
From the weight of snow
Twigs and leaves they take
Cold ice to show

My inner voice
Beckoning to listen
Forging a choice
Why can't I question?

Dan, Kayla, and Brandon came to visit me in the psych unit on Christmas Day. My dad sent lamb, potatoes, and carrots with them. We had a Christmas feast in my room, and we opened presents. Dr. Clark also came to visit. My depression was so acute that I laid on the bed most of the time in a stupor. I hated for my children to see me in such a state.

I was still manic when they released me. This was the darkest time of all but I have a blessed forgetfulness about most of it. The medications calmed the mania but left me extremely drowsy; staying awake to hold a conversation past eight was pointless. My concentration was poor and my memory even worse. Things that I once found so enjoyable—reading, writing, drawing—were impossible. I couldn't make decisions, let alone get out of bed to take the children to school.

Our family was in turmoil, both of us bearing a burden that was difficult to tolerate. After taking Kayla to school, I would come home exasperated and exhausted; in such a state I couldn't take care of the house, make dinners, or get the kids in bed at night. It was frustrating for Dan because he felt like he didn't have a spouse. It seemed that more medicine would only further deaden the facets of my life. This was such a trying time that I'm not sure how Dan stuck in there with me. He is a saint.

My thoughts were equally depressing. I was suicidal. My marriage was falling apart, and the kids could sense that something was wrong. I was convinced that our family would be better off without me. Anxiety over Kayla and Brandon's safety was an obsession. I viewed everyone as if they were going to kidnap them. Kayla was allowed to stay on the front porch only when the door was open.

The side effects of the combination of medications prescribed for me were not easily managed. It was torturous to lay in bed, night after night of interrupted sleep. The nights restless, staring at the ceiling, making friends with the ceiling and the walls. Eyes holding the light from the shadowy moon. Nothing could break the cycle… night after night.

Sleep evading the night
To elude the sanity of sight
Escaping my reality
To find sanity

The lithium caused unquenchable thirst. Even after Dr. Clark's suggestion to suck on a washcloth at night, I couldn't. I would get up, go the bathroom, drink 32 ounces of water and go to bed. This would happen up to five times a night. Sometimes, I would lock myself in the walk-in closet, thinking it was the bathroom, and urinate on the floor. Despite feeling for the door handle, I couldn't find it. I panicked and banged on the door so my husband could let me out. Night after night I would wet my clothes or the bed. Even with the light on I couldn't find the toilet. Most nights I was so drugged I didn't even know that I had to go to the bathroom. It was humiliating and disgusting and I wasn't prepared for this. However, mania is so frightening that even these side-effects were more tolerable.

The wake/sleep cycle would continue all night long and as I fell further away from a restful night's sleep I descended deeper and deeper into the swirling darkness and the fearsome void. The days were long, the nights hauntingly longer; I dreaded waking up each day. Most people have a normal fear of death, but I never felt more depressed than when I wanted those fears to become a reality. It felt so close that I could almost feel it. And it scared me. I felt as if my soul were in a glass case, and everyone could see my every action. *Could they see right through me? My inadequacies, my frailties, my depression, my state of mind? The anxiety. The paranoia. The delusions. The irrationality.*

My head spun in circles trying to find a relief from the hell that I was experiencing and the hell I was putting my family through. In the darkness of the night I reached for my last and final hope; I called Dr. Clark and I took myself off of Lithium. Dr. Clark called me back in the silence of the night, and this became my only lifeline.

Lithium works well for many and is probably the most frequently prescribed medication for bipolar, but we are all a different chemical mix. It is difficult to find the correct dosage of medication for each individual and is generally a trial by error. We all react to various medications or combinations in a different way. I feel blessed that through careful observation Dr. Clark and I have found the correct regime for me. I can't thank him enough. All of my side effects subsided after discontinuing the Lithium, which caused a dramatic change in my memory, concentration, and hand tremors. Dr. Clark stated, "It has been amazingly helpful. I would not have predicted it." The replacement medication Dr. Clark prescribed has finally given sanity and life back to me and I haven't been in the hospital since.

Our Last Trial

"The deeper that sorrow cuts into your being, the more joy you can contain."

~Khalil Gibran, The Prophet

The last trial regarding Kayla's health was when she had a spinal fusion for scoliosis on June 4, 2008, at age nine due to a 55-degree curve in her back. Dan admitted her to surgery at 4:45 a.m. and stayed with her. We had decided it would be better for me to stay home and keep busy. The surgeon made an incision along her spinal cord from the base of her neck to her tailbone, then detached the muscle from the spinal cord on both sides of her spine. Two rods were screwed in, one on each side, with 25 screws to hold them in place. The surgery lasted more than six hours and was highly successful.

Dan called me from the hospital when it was over and after I arrived we were allowed back in the waiting area. They hadn't taken the tube out of her airway, and thoughts of her previous intubations flooded my memory. Her face was puffy and her throat dry from the tube placed in her airway, so she couldn't talk. She didn't recognize us and we hardly recognized her. That was the most difficult for me, and I took it personally. Her earlier hospitalization, just nine years earlier, haunted me, and my faith faltered right before my eyes. Dan seemed to have more compassion and understanding for Kayla. I felt guilty for not being there for the six hours she was in surgery.

Later that day, she was transferred to the sixth floor. The rehabilitation therapists came often to help her get out of bed. They helped her sit up in bed, and she practiced sitting in a chair ten to fifteen minutes at a time. This seemed like an impossible task, and they were going to discharge her after five days! After a few days, she started eating popcorn shrimp, mashed potatoes, and ice cream. I knew she was feeling a lot better because her appetite increased. On the second day, she used the toilet for the first time since her surgery. We held her under her arms and then gently sat her on the toilet. This was painful for her, and we would have to continue it at home. On the third day, the therapists had her in a wheelchair, and Dan often took her on walks through the gardens outside the hospital. After their long walks they went inside the cafeteria, and she ate ice cream with M&Ms.

The days were long, with Kayla at home on the couch, and I had little hope that she would ever get her bubbly personality back. I missed my dear Kayla, and hoped against hope that she would return to the cheerful little girl I knew so well. Dan spent the nights at Kayla's bedside, then I would relieve him in the morning and he would leave for work. During those long days it was difficult to believe that life would be normal again. Visitors came and went, providing comfort in my concern and care for Kayla. My mom came to the hospital and took my place one night because I needed to take my medicine in order to get to bed by 8:30. Although I felt like Kayla needed me by her side, I was torn; I longed to stay there, and I longed for relief. On the fourth day they had her "walking" down the hallway. She couldn't put any pressure on her feet and was literally held up while she walked. The therapist convinced me that she would be able to walk, even up the stairs. On the fifth day, Kayla was walking with help and walked up three steps in the rehabilitation room.

She came home that day and was confined to the couch for the next couple of weeks. During this time we watched a bird's nest with four eggs to see if they would hatch. We took a mirror and held it in such a way as to see inside the nest without touching it. Kayla looked every day to see if the baby birds had hatched; it was therapeutic for her and helped divert attention to something other than the pain in her back. The mama bird kept a close eye on her babies and we tried to stay away from the eggs. The babies hatched and one by one they were pushed from the nest. During this time our good friend Chris visited Kayla often, and Kayla walked the half-mile loop around the neighborhood with him holding her under her arms. The sunshine and fresh air also seemed to lift her spirits. Every day, I would take her up the street to visit Rosie, a golden retriever.

In order for her to get into a standing position she would swing her legs in a 90-degree angle and push her trunk up with her arms. Getting to the bathroom was just as difficult as sitting on the toilet. She would fall back into our arms and then bend at the waist. I wasn't sure she would ever be able to do this alone. She couldn't dress herself without pain. However, miracles do happen! She learned how to get jeans on without bending her back. She would loosen her pant leg, cross her left ankle over her right leg, and quickly put her leg through the pant hole. For three months she was forbidden to jump rope, ride a bike, or jump on a trampoline. She has beaten the odds. She has known pain and now personifies joy.

Serenity

"Being deeply loved by someone gives you strength; loving someone deeply gives you courage."

~Lao-tzu

Our marriage has been solidified and strengthened by having gone through the fire together. We enjoy one another's company once again and life is more lighthearted. I often catch Dan glancing at me in ways that say "I love you." Dan and I have walked where very few have traveled and our journey has led us full circle, a promise that never ends. We never would have dreamed what was ahead for us and how deeply we could love, and how deeply we could suffer, both because of our ill children and my illness. We are now able to take time out for ourselves, and have started dating and holding meaningful conversations, whereas before I couldn't think of things to say, I was so depressed. My concentration and memory had been so poor, and understanding and following a storyline such an impossibility, that books, movies, and conversations were out of the question. I had no interest in anything.

I believe that now he looks forward to being home with me and the children. It was difficult for him to travel and have confidence that our children were safe when I was in no condition to take care of them due to a manic or depressed state. I'm convinced that the only way he could leave for a few days on a business trip was because he exercised faith in the Lord to take care of all of us.

We no longer feel as if we are making our way in dense fog through dangerous waters. Life had been dark and depressing. The only thing that kept us together was our faith and our marriage where we covenanted with one another for eternity. However, he had hope that life would be better and the memories of our wedding day and his faith in me and the Savior would be lasting. Our hopes and dreams consisted of healthy children, financial security, my good health, and a mission to China, which all seem realizable now.

Although our trials and tribulations that we have gone through have stretched us almost to the breaking point, they have solidified our marriage. It is so strong now that I don't believe anything could shake our confidence in one another. The love we feel for one another has developed into a more godly love, a love that goes beyond the grave and reaches far into the heavens. It is a deep trust in one another and a knowledge that life continues on despite our adversities.

It is difficult for me to look from the outside to the inside. My husband has endured more than anyone could imagine. Although I've found this illness to be intensely difficult to live with, it is equally trying to watch someone you love go through it. His love for me may have wavered, but he has never given up on me. However, his frustrations are real and are with merit. Despite all my shortcomings, Dan is extremely forgiving.

Our children are the most important aspect of our lives, and they have been blessed as well by my improved health. I have more self-assurance to define their roles and set limits for both Brandon and Kayla, which in turn makes them feel safer. Before, I was indecisive and anxious. They naturally picked up on this.

Before I quit taking Lithium, I took my medicine at eight o'clock at night and needed to go to bed at 8:30. If Kayla wasn't ready for bed, I would be exhausted and rush her through her nighttime routine: brushing her teeth, combing her hair, reading scriptures, and saying prayers. My weariness was not only noticeable to me, but it put her in a tailspin; oftentimes she would rupture into fits of aggression, flailing her arms and melting to the floor. I pushed her very hard so that I could get to bed on time, which meant we generally accomplished nothing, and I sent her to bed without her nightly routine. Now that I'm no longer taking Lithium, I take my medicine at 8:30 and try to have her in bed by nine. I don't feel drugged anymore and am able to help her accomplish her nightly routine with patience and kindness.

In the morning I had a difficult time getting up, often sleeping in until seven o'clock. Our morning routine was rushed as well, and most of the time she wouldn't respond to me so she was consistently late for school. My frustration with her erupted into her frustration with me. I now get up at 6:30 a.m. and allow her a little time to wake up and then get her into the bathtub. She is self-directed and needs very little encouragement to get ready for school. Life is peaceful, and my love and patience for her has grown immensely.

During the darkest times, Brandon's grades were poor. He wasn't reaching his potential, and I had a difficult time monitoring his homework. He now attends an International Baccalaureate magnet school for the gifted and talented and scored a 140 on his IQ test and ranks in the ninety-ninth percentile. My illness had a negative impact on his education, but he is now excelling in school once again.

Kayla's temper tantrums are fewer and farther between, although she still struggles in many areas. The consequences of my inability to discipline her at that time has led to her unpredictable behavior. She also demonstrates poor impulse control, and it becomes a daily challenge for her to control her intense emotions. It is difficult and demanding for me, and I'm forced to exercise the utmost patience. She is in the Integrated Learning Center (ILC) and is mainstreamed into her fourth-grade class. Although she received occupational, physical, and speech therapy as a toddler, she still struggles in academics. Most of the time she is a well-adjusted little girl and has an exuberance for life. She, too, is a delight.

At one time both Brandon's and Kayla's health was delicate, and our worry over them consumed us. The fear of losing both of them was a constant reminder of how very fragile life is for all of us. We never know when our time is up. The Lord has given us extra time with these two souls; they are truly gifts from Him. Every day we kneel in prayer as a family; we are grateful for the good health our children enjoy, as well as for my health. We have been tremendously blessed.

It's been more than five years since my last hospitalization. With the correct balance of medications (which for me is Risperdal, Lamictal and Clozapine), my life has been completely stabilized. I no longer feel as dependent on Dr. Clark as I once did, and I do not see him as often. Now that I no longer take Lithium my hand tremors are completely gone. My ability to draw, write and seek spiritual strength has returned, along with my cognitive abilities. And my faith is strong. I feel life stirring in the depths of my being. I like the person I've become as a result of the refiner's fire; and if you ask me who I am, I might even remember me! I never could have attempted to write this story without the right medications for me; it has transformed my life completely.

Even if I'm not the slender girl of my college years, I like what I see in the mirror now. My weight had been a huge battle for me due to medication, depression, and two pregnancies. The size of my jeans doubled from a size 12 to a size 28. I was incredibly low spirited and felt both hopeless and worthless. Dan always made me feel beautiful, even when I knew I wasn't. Kristin never gave up on me. She came over every day in the winter weather to walk with me on the Highline Canal. We walked—rain, snow, or sunshine. I would never guess that I would lose those extra pounds only to gain most of them back again before finally returning to a normal weight.

My success in losing weight came from Weight Watchers. I lost more than 120 pounds in three years. I was zealous about attending meetings and "weighing in" each week. I had support from an exceptional leader, Betsy, who encouraged me at my highest weight and lowest point. Every day for over an hour I worked out on my treadmill. The athletic abilities developed in my youth enabled me to exercise on a consistent basis, with determination and intensity, making weight loss possible.

At this time in my life I really love who I am and feel more beautiful today for the road I've traveled than ever before. I have become the woman I've always longed to be, creating a home, and taking care of my children.

I have a completely positive outlook on life. Our prayers have been answered and it is our belief that life will continue in normalcy. The Lord's unconditional love for me has allowed me to walk on the bright side once again. We are optimistic that the current regime of medicines will continue allowing me to maintain a life that is conducive to raising a family and being a competent partner in marriage.

Although at times we felt discouraged by our obstacles, we now view them as stepping stones to a better reality. Our lives, once diverted by heart-wrenching circumstances, have now converged. We have attained the serenity you reach when you've been to the very end, beyond hope, and yet made it back.

Even though bipolar never goes away completely, with the proper treatment a person with bipolar can live a normal life and prevent relapses. Although I will continue to need medication, I feel rescued from the ups and downs. The intense uphill climb has been replaced by a more moderate road that winds back and forth, slightly up and down, to create an interesting journey. I had often found myself off the beaten path and walking barefoot among the thistles and thorns to escape the burning heat of the paved road. I realize that my life will include some u-turns, forks in the road, and one-way streets, as will all of our lives.

The direction I've taken has prompted self-reflection. A stone thrashed by a swift, tumbling river becomes chiseled and, eventually smooth. I feel I've been this stone. In the downward spiraling of this illness, I've found myself chiseled and smoothed by God's guiding hand, a force greater than myself. My feelings of insecurity, anxiety, and self-doubt have been replaced by greater self-assurance and empathy for others.

My failures and successes have helped me to understand humanity as I reflect on my own life. I pray I no longer exemplify the person I was but the person I can be. My trust and love in the Savior has developed in the depths of my being as I have relied on Him to carry me through my nightmare journey, and I hope and pray that reading about my journey will help carry you through yours. It is a double-edged life.